LIVING RECOVERY

LIVING RECOVERY

Youth Speak Out on "Owning"
Mental Illness

JoAnn Elizabeth Leavey

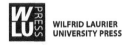

**WILFRID LAURIER
UNIVERSITY PRESS**

Wilfrid Laurier University Press acknowledges the financial support of the Government of Canada through the Canada Book Fund for our publishing activities.

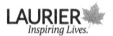 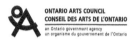

Library and Archives Canada Cataloguing in Publication

Leavey, JoAnn Elizabeth, [date], author
    Living recovery : youth speak out on "owning" mental illness / JoAnn Elizabeth Leavey.

Includes bibliographical references and index.
Issued in print and electronic formats.
ISBN 978-1-55458-917-3 (pbk.).—ISBN 978-1-55458-918-0 (pdf).—
ISBN 978-1-55458-919-7 (epub)

    1. Youth—Mental health. 2. Youth—Interviews. 3. Mentally ill—Interviews. 4. Stigma (Social psychology). I. Title.

RJ503.L42 2015   616.8900835   C2014-905571-4
                                             C2014-905572-2

Cover design by David Drummond. Front-cover image: Shutterstock_56396311. Text design by Lime Design Inc..

© 2015 Wilfrid Laurier University Press
Waterloo, Ontario, Canada
www.wlupress.wlu.ca

This book is printed on FSC® certified paper and is certified Ecologo. It contains post-consumer fibre, is processed chlorine free, and is manufactured using biogas energy.

Printed in Canada

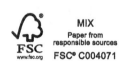

MIX
Paper from
responsible sources
FSC® C004071

CONTENTS

THREE

Youth Participants: Who Are They? 43

FOUR

Youth Speak: Mental Health Experiences and Needs 55

FIVE

Understanding: Integrating the Results 125

SIX

Where Are We and Where Do We Go from Here? 145

ACKNOWLEDGEMENTS

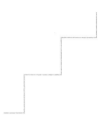

THIS BOOK IS THE RESULT of several years of research, clinical work, advocacy, systems reviews, systems planning, evaluation, and discussion on the topic of youth and mental illness/wellness. Many local and international clinical and research colleagues have inspired me to further my studies and research in patient/client-centred work in order to continue to create and offer perspectives in a best practices environment. Others have also inspired me over my career, including the many patients, clients, youth, and advocacy groups for mental health services whom I have had the great pleasure to serve. They have been a constant source of information and have willingly participated in my research to better the clinical practice environment for those individuals with newly emerging mental health challenges. For this I am grateful and thankful, as research, and in particular qualitative research, helps us to continuously evolve better and promising clinical practices.

I would like to extend special thanks to Gordon Cone and the staff at New Outlook, Toronto, Ontario; Dr. Patrick McGorry, John Moran, and the staff at ORYGEN, Melbourne, Australia; and Dr. Mary Moller, Dr. Michael Rice, and the late Donna Androsky at the Suncrest Wellness Centre, Spokane, Washington, who facilitated my acceptance as a researcher with their youth clients at their respective youth or person-centred, community-based mental health programs. Without their collective insights, assistance, and support, this research would not have been possible.

Particular thanks go to all of the youth in Australia, the United States, and Canada who gave thoughtful and powerful interviews regarding their lives and their experiences with mental health problems. In some cases, participants were facing multiple challenges, but without exception, they wanted to contribute to furthering our understanding of youth and the experience of living with mental illness.

I would like to thank Dr. Margaret Schneider, Dr. Jeanne Watson, Dr. Lana Stermac, and Dr. Francis G. Hare for their encouragement, assistance, and constructive and insightful criticism with my previous research on youth and mental health. My thanks also go to Judge Marvin Zuker for his genuine and excellent work with children and families and his interest in research that continues to evolve and enlighten clinical practice with the hope of helping children and families live productive, safe, and satisfying lives. All collectively encouraged me to further my research and complete this book.

Thank you to Mayne Ellis for transcribing all 53 interviews. I was impressed with her ability to adapt to different accents and so accurately transcribe what was said. Thanks are definitely in order to my editors, Jacqueline Larson, Janet Money, and Janice Dyer, who provided editing and expert editing advice.

I would like to acknowledge the constant support, encouragement, and practical assistance of family, friends, and colleagues in Vancouver, Toronto, Melbourne, Australia, and Washington State, without which this work would have been much more difficult to complete.

Finally, I would like to acknowledge the wonderful resilience of the youth interviewed in this study by providing a quote from one participant that sums up and describes their collective wisdom and learned self-empowerment:

"I own the illness; the illness does not own me."

ONE

Framing the Context for Youth Living with Mental Illness

Introduction

E SPECIALLY IN QUALITATIVE RESEARCH, it is important and necessary for researchers to be located in the research to ensure that any bias is uncovered and evident. The following information describes that location. I have worked in the mental health field for over fifteen years as a clinician, researcher, administrator, educator, and policy-maker. I have always been genuinely interested in people's mental and medical health, social stories, and recovery. When working with patients (especially with young people ages 16 to 24), over time I came to see the importance of early intervention. It was a key component in avoiding or at least mitigating some of the social stigma and social losses caused by having a chronic mental health condition. In addition, early intervention helped youth avoid some of the physical and emotional effects of their condition.

Inspired by these observations, I decided to start researching early intervention and stigma in the area of first episode psychosis. The information I gathered underscored my clinical observation that early intervention resulted in better outcomes for individuals, especially for young people experiencing mental health problems. What I did not initially see was a great deal of research focusing on the voices of the youth themselves. Since then, however, there has been an explosion of research focusing on early intervention, including a strong emphasis on young people. Yet there is still a gap in terms of what youth themselves have to say about their experiences with mental illness (Caine & Boydell, 2010).

This book is part of a growing body of research literature that supports reducing stigma, listening to individuals who live with mental health problems as experts in their experiences, and focusing on best practices to help them with recovery. This book focuses on the experiences of youth and provides a way of understanding mental illness/health in terms of the categories of ELAR: *Emergence* of a problem, *Loss* of self and social standing, *Adaptation* to a new understanding of self and other, and *Recovery* from a mental illness process.

In conducting this research, it was my privilege to hear fifty-three young people from three countries describe to me their journeys with mental illness. Together we explored what it was like living with a mental health problem; their subsequent adjustment problems due to the social stigma associated with mental illness; how they became alienated or self-marginalized because of the symptoms of the illness; and the social consequences they experienced because of the stigma. The youth were excited to have the opportunity to share their stories and express what was important to them about their experiences. They were firmly committed to telling their stories so that newly diagnosed youth or those beginning to feel "different" from the norm would have a chance to know that others feel the same way. The youth also wanted to encourage a more generous understanding of mental illness, one that includes less judgment and stigma. They opened their hearts so that others would open their minds to reduce negative labels and stigma. It is with this aim that I share their stories.

I would like to start by explaining my interest in young people experiencing mental health problems. As a result of several years of research, clinical work, advocacy, systems reviews, systems planning, evaluation, and discussion on the topic of youth and mental illness/wellness, I was impressed by the positive contributions that young people made to their own adaptation and recovery processes. I was particularly interested in their resilience in the face of being labelled with a mental health problem. For instance, these youth still managed to contribute to society, even though they felt stigmatized and initially frightened by the process of receiving a diagnosis and intervention.

Further, I was impressed by their complete willingness to enhance our understanding by bravely sharing their stories. Their goal was to help other youth who might not be receiving the support they needed, or who were experiencing their first episode or emergence of a mental health problem and did not know whom to turn to. Finally, these young people were concerned about the future and were steadfastly working toward both personal and societal/community goals. All of these factors attracted my interest and curiosity.

In this book, you will learn how youth experience the emergence of their mental illness, the losses they experience, and how they adapt and recover. This information has the potential to open dialogue between youth, care providers, administrators, and policy-makers with the goal of developing a system of care that is more youth-centred. When mental health care programs and services become more relevant, timely, and meaningful, they then become more effective in the recovery process for young people.

So open your minds and your hearts to what is being presented. Use this information to help young people—or anyone you may encounter who is experiencing a mental health problem—to feel more accepted in society. Give them a chance to recover from the real problem, not the subsequent social marginalization they experience from being labelled as "different." It will take courage to stand up to old norms and advocate for young people with mental health problems. Reading this book will help convince you of the tremendous courage, strength, and insights these youth have regarding their own experiences, along with their desire to share in order to help other youth. This book is about their journeys, their experiences, and their offer to teach us what they know; their ultimate hope is that we will listen and that others will suffer less.

....

Terms Used in This Book

■ THE WORLD HEALTH ORGANIZATION (WHO) defines mental health as "a state of well-being in which the individual realises his or her own abilities, can cope with the normal stresses of life, can work productively and fruitfully, and is able to make a contribution to his or her community" (2001, p. 1). The Public Health Agency of Canada also has a broad definition: "Mental health is the capacity of each and all of us to feel, think and act in ways that enhance our ability to enjoy life and deal with the challenges we face. It is a positive sense of emotional and spiritual well-being that respects the importance of culture, equity, social justice, interconnections and personal dignity" (2006, p. 2). I use the terms mental health problem, mental illness, and mental disorder interchangeably due to the inconsistent definitions and application of the terms in the available literature, among mental health workers, and by the participants themselves.

The participants in this research self-identified a wide range of conditions that they labelled as mental illness, including depression, psychosis, bipolar disorder, schizophrenia, anxiety disorder, post-traumatic stress syndrome, obsessive-compulsive disorder, personality disorders, eating disorders, learning disabilities, delusional disorder, mood disorder, generalized anxiety disorder, and Asperger syndrome. For the purposes of this book, all of these conditions are considered to be a mental illness.

Finally, I use the terms youth, young people, transition-aged youth, and transitional youth interchangeably. Further, the terms transitional youth and transition-aged youth refer to youth in transition through the developmental stages from adolescence to young adulthood.

············

Who Is This Book For?

■ A DIAGNOSIS OF MENTAL ILLNESS can be incorporated into daily living by considering mental illness as "just" another problem rather than something to be feared or stigmatized. The information provided in this book will help youth, parents, health care providers, policy-makers, governments, and service systems to understand mental illness in a different way. Appropriate and effective early intervention (in particular, medication) to help stabilize the illness so that youth can concentrate on reclaiming their social and identity losses is an important first step. Staying with their families when possible (as opposed to institutionalization) may help youth stabilize during their recovery and rehabilitation. Health care providers, policy-makers, governments, and service systems need to begin to address service delivery needs based in part on the psychosocial development of youth. Service provision needs to be developmentally focused so that youth can meet their life cycle needs; this means providing them with the opportunity to rehabilitate, to get work-related training and education, and to access organized support. Such supports include peer-related activities, groups, and programs. These peer groups need to include advocacy; they also need to educate individuals and the community and facilitate the recovery and reintegration of youth.

The identified gaps in service systems for youth with mental health problems need attention, but without formal peer support services for youth, services are less effective. When formal psychosocial supports and services with formalized peer components are available, more potential exists for youth to use these programs as an avenue of access to formal treatment interventions and as the basis for maintaining ongoing recovery.

....

Redefining Our Understanding of Mental "Illness"

■ OUR UNDERSTANDING of what mental illness means to youth can be expressed as follows:

Illness is a process that helps us understand the experience of youth who have been diagnosed with a mental illness. We can view this process as a series of stages—emergence, loss, adaptation, and recovery—that youth move through during their illness. Understanding the onset of mental illness in young people as a process is an important avenue by which to approach how youth adapt and change in relation to their internal and external circumstances of biological and social change.

Overall, youth with mental illness experience their social world as a place where they are labelled and stigmatized. Youth with mental illness are placed in a position where they must negotiate the world *through* mental illness, which is present in all aspects of their internal physiological and external social experiences. The meaning of their world has been created by the social and biological reality of mental illness, which defines their internal and external environments. Therefore, what they experience externally has the potential to be expressed internally through a developmental disruption. Youth experience the effects of the social construction of mental illness and subsequently may experience the reality of an "interrupted self." A self who has been interrupted by mental illness has a negative identity, and this has implications for social maturation and life-stage development. This social reality is further complicated by young people having no control over the biological fact that they have acquired the illness. Therefore, initially youth are victim to their illness both biologically and socially and must learn how to cope with this reality state, or way of being, and recover.

The underlying thesis of this book is that mental illness does not define the person—rather, it is part of what that person must cope with. Mental wellness or health is the integration of this knowledge so that the youth can embrace life as a person, not a mentally ill individual.

....

The Journey of Youth Through the Mental Health System

■ THERE IS LITTLE RESEARCH about young people's stories of their experiences with mental illness. The research that is available expresses the deep and complex understanding that youth often have about their lives (Caine & Boydell, 2010). For example, "the youth we listened to do not necessarily describe themselves as victims, but as imaginative, creative, and resourceful human beings with social, cultural, and political agency" (Clandinin et al., 2010). These researchers emphasize the importance of listening to youth as a way to learn more about how we can help; the focus is on inquiry rather than on finding solutions.

Other researchers have focused on understanding how and why youth seek help for mental health difficulties (Santor, Kusumakar, Poulin, & LeBlanc, 2007). In this school-based research project, female students, more depressed students, and those with more severe mood problems were more likely to use an Internet-based program to obtain information and then to visit school health centres and guidance counsellors.

Framing the Context for Youth Living with Mental Illness

Alex: *I just feel that I'm sad that I have a mental illness, because, well, for one thing I'm just sad because I don't want something bad. I see mental illness as bad, a bad omen, and especially since society used mental illness as something crazy or disturbed people have. Like they have those TV movies where, you know, a person is compulsively doing this and they're thinking about spiders and spiders crawl on them. They make it so drastic, these illnesses, that people see it just as bad.*[1]

Mental illness is a social illness, as much as if not more than a biological illness. In fact, the social effect of mental illness is often more difficult to deal with than the illness itself. This chapter examines the impact of a mental illness diagnosis on youth, including the idea that with mental illness, we are really fighting stigma. The chapter also reviews the needs of transition-aged youth, explores the concept of metaphor and mental illness, and reviews the social construction of mental illness. This is a critical chapter for practitioners in terms of how they think about and respond to youth presenting with mental health problems.

....

The Effects of a Mental Illness Diagnosis on Youth

Stigma

As a mental health care practitioner, I have listened to accounts of the battles people have experienced while recovering from serious mental illnesses. I have observed that the most prevalent issue in recovery, whether the person is a youth or an adult, is dealing with the social effects of the associated stigma related to the term "mental illness." Dealing with this stigma is the hardest part of recovery. A mental illness diagnosis, in essence, means

---

1   Note that all identifying factors have been removed from participant quotes, including country of origin, to respect participant privacy and for identity protection.

acquiring a label that potentially "sentences" a person to the burden of acquiring a "social disorder." The research in this field supports the view that the social effects of mental illness are at times more difficult to deal with than the illness itself. As a result, coping with mental illness in some ways has more to do with addressing and enduring the stigma, discrimination, and prejudice that accompany it (Davidson, 2003; Leavey, 2003, 2005; Moller & Murphy, 1997; Rice & Moller, 2006; Wahl, 1999). In addition, stigma about seeking help creates barriers to help-seeking for mental health problems (Gulliver, Griffiths, & Christensen, 2010). In essence, having a mental health problem is social, emotional, psychological, familial, and biological.

When young people living with mental health problems talk about their mental illness and its social effects, they are usually talking about prejudice and the effects of being labelled and marginalized because of mental illness. Because of being "different," a person acquires a social illness that leads to rejection, rather than a sympathetic and medical response free of judgment. To grasp the magnitude of the social, psychological, cultural, and economic impact of being labelled a sociably undesirable person, I have provided some basic operational definitions that lead groups to define behaviour as socially undesirable or unacceptable (Aronson, Wilson, & Akert, 2005):

> *Prejudice.* A widespread phenomenon present in all societies of the world. Social psychologists define prejudice as a hostile or negative attitude toward a distinguishable group of people based solely on their group membership.

> *Stereotype.* The cognitive component of the prejudiced attitude; it is defined as a generalization about a group whereby identical characteristics are assigned to virtually all members, regardless of actual variation among the members.

> *Discrimination.* The behavioural component of the prejudiced attitude; is defined as an unjustified negative or harmful action toward members of a group based on their membership in that group.

Youth describe being ostracized from their peer group because they have been negatively stereotyped. As a result, they are socially placed in the margins. Unfortunately, such stereotypes seem acceptable in modern culture. One youth described how Hollywood often equates mental illness or mental difference with words such as mad, crazy, loony, nuts, and so on. The mass media have the power to produce a particular image of mental illness, which then affects what we aspire to and how we comply with social norms (Lasch, 1979; Sontag, 1977). The media also influence how we decide who is "in" and who and what is "out"—that is, how we decide what is "appropriate" (Lasch, 1979). Negative statements by the non-ill play into how people with illness ultimately are treated in daily life.

Social stigma arises when an individual is disqualified from full social acceptance (Goffman, 1963). Group behaviour and social functioning are essential elements in the evolutionary process of social integration and maturity. Groups work to promote their members, and when one member becomes a threat, the individual is stigmatized and becomes an outcast. Researchers indicate that "because group life benefits from an understanding of and adherence to accepted rules and scripts for coordinated action and interaction, individuals seen as unpredictable (e.g., people labelled with certain mental illnesses) are likely to be stigmatized" (Neuberg, Smith, & Asher, 2000, p. 46). Individuals with mental illness are seen as having "blemishes of character" (Biernat & Dovidio, 2000, p. 88). Those who have infectious diseases or mental illnesses such as schizophrenia are stigmatized, excluded, and avoided. Group members may avoid persons with a "spoiled identity" (Goffman, 1963) because of the fear of stigma by association (Neuberg et al., as cited in Heatherton et al., 2000) or, as Goffman coined it, "courtesy stigma."

Negative Portrayal of Mental Illness

In North American society today, people with mental illness are represented in negative and stereotypical ways and are portrayed as violent, weird, sick, mad, dangerous, and worthless (Crumpton, Weinstein, Acker, & Annis, 1967, as cited in Heatherton et al., 2000; Scheff, 1966, as cited in Heatherton et al., 2000). This portrayal only compounds the problem of social acceptance and understanding; and ultimately it compromises our ability to destigmatize and demystify mental illness.

This socio-cultural view of mental illness is critical to how young people with a mental illness see themselves and their role in society. If they cannot find positive images of themselves or receive encouraging feedback from their peer groups, building or rebuilding a healthy sense of self becomes an onerous task. Instead of being enabled to seek help and recover, with social support to do so, young people may be tempted to conceal or disguise their mental illness (Goffman, 1963). Members of stigmatized groups may also try sometimes to pass as members of non-stigmatized groups. This includes people who are homosexual, persons with a mental disorder or physical illness, or those simply considered different (Cole, Kemeny, & Taylor, 1997, as cited in Heatherton et al., 2000).

Understanding Stigma from a Frame Analysis

Goffman's (1974) theory of frame analysis helps us understand the stigma that youth with mental illness experience. He describes two kinds of frameworks: natural frameworks, which deal with the natural occurrence of purely physical events such as weather and climate, which humans do not control; and social frameworks, which deal with those events or parts of events that occur through human wilfulness, purpose, goal seeking, and manipulation. In natural frameworks, events happen singly, from start to finish, because of natural determinants, which Goffman calls "unguided doings." Some agency is implied—there is a subjection to social appraisal that views the action based on its honesty, outcome, elegance, and so forth. In contrast, the events in social frameworks are referred to as "guided doings." The consequences of guided doings are continually monitored, and when things are not on track, special compensatory effort is needed (Goffman, 1974). Natural physical events cannot be controlled; social doings *can* be controlled. For example, for the most part we cannot control getting cancer or having a heart attack, but it is perceived that we can control an angry outburst, mental distress (e.g., just get over it), or anxiety.

Goffman considered that society makes significant assumptions about events by way of the "astounding complex." "In our society," he says, "the very significant assumption is generally made that all events—without exception—can be contained and managed within the conventional system of beliefs. We tolerate the unexplained but not the inexplicable" (Goffman, 1974, p. 30). This interpretative method is part of a primary framework, which means that once events are recognized, we analyze and interpret them through particular schemata. Frame analysis provides a fresh view on mental illness. When considering natural and social events taken together from this perspective, we can see stigma and the phenomenon of mental illness in a new light. For example, in Goffman's astounding complex, individuals are required to interpret an event that is outside of their conventional system of beliefs, such as witnessing the emergence of mental illness in a friend. The individual may understand the emergence of the mental illness as not his peer's fault. He may interpret the event from a primary frame, seeing the illness as an unguided doing, the invisible part of the problem. However, he might interpret the ensuing behaviours, the visible part, as guided doings because behaviour outside the norm (outside convention) is usually seen as something that can be controlled.

It is difficult enough for young people to grow up and deal with the biology, psychology, and challenges of attaining milestones of social and economic achievement. But for young people who have been labelled with a social disorder, their difference or distance from "normal" ends for them any possibility of being part of the in-group. Goffman describes this in-group/out-group as part of his "astounding complex": the individual may be seen by his or her peers as having fallen victim to mental illness and therefore not be blamed, for it is "not the peer's fault." However, the peer's resulting behaviours may be seen as controllable, and therefore the peer group assigns blame to the victim of mental illness since she is not controlling her behaviours, which are clearly outside group norms (Goffman, 1974).

The mentally ill person thus becomes the victim of the illness (the purely physical unguided doing) but at the same time is held responsible for any behaviours arising from the illness, which are viewed as wilful acts (guided behaviours) (Goffman, 1974). Stigma results when peers and friends back away from what they see as the mentally ill person's wilful acts. The peer group of a youth with a mental illness can understand mental illness only from their own developmental stage. They are going through their own developmental identity and intimacy crises, and thus they may not be able to cope with difference or oddness. They typically see the behaviours as unexplained and the person exhibiting them as responsible.

We can use frame analysis theory to understand mental illness in two ways: the illness itself is a physical frame or unguided doing that affects an individual; and the behavioural aspects of the illness, because they are visible to others as unconventional behaviour, are controllable (guided doings). Herein lies the contradictory foundation of stigma—peers may understand that an individual has fallen victim to an illness for which no blame or judgment is attached, but the resulting behavioural activity is judged and stigmatized. The behaviour is not attached to the victim; rather, it is seen as attached to a person who is in control of his behaviour(s) (Goffman, 1974).

Labelling

Stigmatization is the process of labelling behaviour as deviant (Heatherton et al., 2000). Part of this process lies in how groups behave, determine norms, and decide what is "deviant." Whatever group exists in a particular context will determine what is acceptable behaviour and what is not. In general, this is part of a group's function, and the existing group defines the label's context (Heatherton et al., 2000). The socio-cultural reaction to being labelled is considered, in part, a way of explaining how behaviours may be seen as deviant (Becker, 1973). If a person is labelled with something that has an associated stigma, the associated stigma may become a catalyst for the person "becoming" or adopting the label itself through a process of self-fulfilling prophecy. In other words, the individual may be at risk for actualizing the label as a result of group pressure or group projection.

Individuals also learn from one another by keeping "an eye on what others have done, are doing, and may do" (Becker, 1973, p. 82). It is typical in-group behaviour for individuals to figure out how they fit in and then adjust to established social norms, and to choose or discern how they would like to be viewed by the group and what they expect or hope to receive back from their group. We could say that both the "labeller" and the "labelled" have subconsciously agreed to their roles. The labeller needs to be viewed by her peers as having some sort of moral authority, and the labelled is in a disadvantaged position because of the disapproved behaviour she is exhibiting (Becker, 1973). This is a broad interpretation of the theory, intended to provide a basic understanding of the role of labelling as it applies to youth mental illness.

Stigmatized people are devalued, ostracized, marginalized, shunned, rejected, assaulted, and insulted. Individuals can and do experience cruelty and hostility because of the stigma of "difference" (Heatherton et al., 2000). When individuals feel marginalized or dispossessed, they can feel a profound lack of worth. Some researchers feel there has been an inadequate amount of attention paid to the "motives, cognitions, and emotional reactions of those being stigmatized, and even less attention ... devoted to analyzing interactions between those who are stigmatized and those doing the stigmatizing" (Heatherton et al., 2000, p. xi).

People with mental illness, the labelled, have an inherent disadvantage based on disapproved behaviours, as demonstrated by the derogatory names assigned to people with a mental problem, such as mental, crazy, weird, not normal, cuckoo, and so on. The labeller in turn may be frightened of deviant or disapproved behaviour, perhaps because he fears becoming these things, running the risk of being ostracized from his current social position. As Goffman observed, "persons who come to the attention of a psychiatrist typically come to the attention of their lay associates first. What psychiatrists see as mental illness, the lay public usually first sees as offensive behaviour ... behaviour worthy of scorn, hostility, and other negative and social sanctions" (Goffman, 1967, p. 137). It is unfortunate that mentally ill people often end up with the intervention of a psychiatrist based on what has been labelled as bad behaviour.

Socialization refers to the external social and cultural influences on people as they go through life: "Every society reproduces its culture, its norms, its underlying assumptions, its modes of organizing experience ... The process of socialization modifies human nature to conform to the prevailing social norms" (Lasch, 1979, p. 34). We can understand development as the "unfolding from within," whereas socialization is a "molding from without" (Levinson, 1980, p. 270). Every social system has a set of processes regarding class, culture, and organization by which its members are influenced and shaped. Normally individuals have many opportunities of membership through their work, family, gender, class, and religion. In addition, each society shapes its members and categorizes their rights and obligations by age and stage. Often there are markers that legitimate the passing from one age and stage to the next. Institutions such as schools, work environments, and places of worship provide and communicate the cultural meanings of various ages and the expectations surrounding the transition and passage into new roles and social status (Levinson, 1980). If a person has acquired the external label and stigma of being "mentally ill," and because of the social images of what is "normal" has internalized this idea of a "spoiled identity" or being outside the norm, the young person may be left with the dual burden of being not only labelled as different but *believing* he is different or abnormal.

Destigmatizing Mental Illness

Imagine breaking your leg and being frightened to go to emergency because negative social stigma was attached to having a broken leg. You would think twice about treatment, and you would not be able to concentrate on what you needed medically for fear of the negative social consequences. Some individuals with broken legs would therefore choose not to be treated and would go on in agony or die from the subsequent physical consequences, such as infection. Now replace the broken leg with mental illness. We need to understand the meaning of stigma if we are to move beyond our societal fears and help young people with mental illnesses to actually focus on the physiological/psychological issues.

Being diagnosed with a mental illness, AIDS, or some other socially undesirable condition can result in stigma that never leaves the person, even if she is restored to near-normal functioning (Lorber, 1997; Sontag, 1978, 1989). "Conversely, patients with severe disabilities, chronic conditions, or terminal illness, if they meet their situation with good grace, stoicism, cheerfulness, and gratitude for care, may be called heroic or saintly" (Lorber, 1997, p. 5). Before illnesses such as cancer, AIDS (Sontag, 1978, 1989), tuberculosis, syphilis, typhoid, and leprosy had treatments that could sustain an acceptable quality of life, the stigma associated with these diseases was greater. Sontag (1989) suggests that by normalizing and integrating diseases such as cancer into our consciousness, we can view them as "just a disease."

We can apply the concept of normalizing and integration to a young person experiencing psychosis or any other mental health problem: rather than seeing that person as having an emotional defect or a life sentence of psychosocial struggle, we should consider a mental health problem to be "just a problem," or "just an illness." The challenge then shifts to whether we can move chronic or severe mental illnesses from a state of stigmatization to a state of normalcy, where they can be fully assimilated or mainstreamed into the broader social experience and perhaps ultimately receive full acceptance. "When searching for the right language" will be irrelevant because "people will have superseded their labels, symptoms and behaviours" (Hamid-Balma, 2005, p. 5), then we will have arrived at the point where mental illness is an accepted illness that a person may happen to have rather than a societal devastation or shameful experience. Sontag (1978, 1989) further suggests that if individuals are unencumbered by stigma and its negative metaphors, they will be freer to approach their problems in a practical and systematic way: "Get doctors to tell you the truth; be an informed active patient; find yourself good treatment because good treatment does exist" (Sontag, 1989, p. 103).

One way of destigmatizing the self is to "eliminate the stigmatizing condition" (Miller & Major, 2000, p. 252). This is an unrealistic task for someone with psychosis or other mental health problems, since individuals do not choose to have a mental illness any more than someone suffering from an addiction or AIDS does. A paradigm shift in how our society views psychosis and other mental health problems may help destigmatize mental illness. It might be that as treatments advance and individuals are able to improve and stabilize, fewer stigmas will be attached to the problem. An increased awareness about young people who suffer from mental illnesses may also help challenge negative stereotypes.

The ultimate goal is to help individuals concentrate on recovery from their illness diagnosis rather than focus their energies on being constantly vigilant about their social status and social acceptance. If this could happen, individuals might have a better chance at receiving early intervention and beginning their processes of recovery, for they would not be afraid to seek out treatment in exchange for social alienation. It is well known that the recovery process is helped when early intervention can be accessed (Malla & Norman, 1999; McGorry, Edwards, Mihalopoulos, Harrigna, & Jackson, 1996).

It is important to understand the in-group/out-group positioning of this age group, for this will give insight into how and why internal and external stigma is created in adolescents. Addressing the developmental needs of both the afflicted person and the affected peer group will generate important insight into the behaviour of stigma, which is expressed as social withdrawal both in the peer group and in the individual experiencing mental illness. This insight could provide some useful direction into what kind of education is needed to decrease stigma in this age group. How can we help reduce the fear of the stigma of mental illness for youth? How can we make the inexplicable explicable? A developmental understanding of both groups—those who create stigma and those who receive it—is required to advance our understanding of why and how stigma is given or delivered and how it is received and experienced. This might help arrest stigma's impact through stigma reduction education about mental illness and its consequential behaviours, thereby reducing the anxiety about the unknown or misunderstood.

Addressing the internal and external social stigma in the context of mental illness and the life stages would allow us to uncover information about the lack of full social integration and acceptance. From a social standpoint, it is vital to understand, predict, and explain the strength of the impact that stigma from mental illness has on this group. The obvious challenge is to understand the degree to which stigma influences an individual's ability to heal, reintegrate, and adapt to his social context. If the essence of stigma means that a person is in a "one down" position with his social counterparts, how does that affect his identity, his sense of self, and his ability to overcome the psychological nature of the disease? Goffman and Jones both state that if the "stigmatized attribute becomes, in the eyes of others, the most important characteristic in judging and responding to the person, it thus pervades all social interactions" (as cited in Wahl, 1999, p. 12).

Self-Marginalization

In addition to being labelled and experiencing loss, youth with mental illness also feel the need to hide their "illness identity" through a process of self-marginalization to protect themselves from the negative social consequences of being labelled "crazy." Mental illness disrupts their lives on every level, but especially their developmental transitions: from childhood to adolescence in some cases, from late adolescence to young adulthood in others. This interruption causes difficulties with self and social identity, as well as with social and maturational development, due to the social effects of marginalization and stigma associated with their illnesses. Smyth insists that youth have been "speaking back from the margins, if only we are able to engage and decipher," and that they will continue to do so (2013). This researcher also emphasizes that youth experiencing mental illness should not be seen as victims or as at risk; rather, they are "active agents exercising choices and making decisions about their lives in situations that amount to 'speaking back'" (Smyth, 2013, p. 43). So it is important to understand what youth go through if we are to help them achieve their life goals, and if we are to address their mental health and social and emotional needs. Further, it is important for us to open our minds to understand that mental illness is secondary to a young person's personhood (or anybody's). Having a mental illness is part of a person's experience, but it need not define that person.

Assessing the effects of mental illness in relation to the critical point of adult identity development requires two efforts: we must explore the role of labelling and stigma for youth in their internal worlds, and we must examine the "meaning" of that role in the external environment. In other words, what effects do internalized stigma, the self-judgment of labelling, and self-imposed aspects of marginalization have on the psychosocial development of youth? Equally, what is the impact of external stigma, marginalization, and labelling? The meaning of mental illness for youth is multi-layered and in a constant state of redefinition and change. So, how does this affect the stabilization process, the ability to heal, and the ability to maintain recovery? Does this dual burden prolong the recovery process? To understand what mental illness "means" to youth, we need to understand how *they* perceive the relationship between their interior and exterior worlds.

All youth need the opportunity to define themselves in order to prepare for adulthood. That includes youth who are living with mental health problems. However, Western society and many cultures around the world view those living with mental health problems with suspicion, often shunning, ostracizing, and ignoring them, and sometimes treating them as criminals or as deserving of punishment. Despite the negative social stigma experienced by young people, and no matter how disenfranchised they feel, they usually learn how to adapt and recover in their respective contexts. The *process* of learned coping and adaptation allows them to gain a sense of wellness and recovery grounded in their own experience and wisdom. What is of greatest concern for young people aged 16 to 27 is the need to manage the transition from adolescence to adulthood *in addition to* adapting to (or chafing against) a negative social label (Erikson, 1980).

....

Youth, Metaphor, and Mental Illness

■ SOCIAL METAPHORS can negatively affect how we interpret mental illness. That interpretation, as well as the choice of language, can determine whether someone is accepted or rejected in a social sense. Using the terminology of mental illnesses to describe negative behaviour has the potential to harm individuals who are actually experiencing those illnesses by condoning stigmatization, in that a label is being used to describe negative behaviours in everyday situations. Sontag (1989) offers an interesting perspective on the use of metaphor in society. She theorizes that society has understood itself through metaphor as far back as Plato and Aristotle, who wrote that "metaphor consists in giving the thing a name that belongs to something else" (as cited in Sontag, 1989, p. 93). Naming a thing as something else is the "spawning ground of most kinds of understanding, including scientific understanding and expressiveness" (Sontag, 1989, p. 93). If society conceives things in terms of metaphors, then clearly, metaphors are extremely powerful and significant in determining how society views particular things.

A person's thinking or relationship to a particular circumstance has the potential to be profoundly altered depending on whether a negative or positive metaphor is used. Some examples: the media often refer to fractured thinking as "schizophrenic"; a politician who makes a mistake is said to be "out of touch with reality" or "delusional"; people who are excited or show exuberance may be referred to as "high on life" or "manic." A colleague of mine was having an internal ethical crisis over layoffs he had to administer. He said he was "not taking his lithium," implying that he was a victim of his circumstances, out of control, angry, perhaps irrational, and certainly "not himself." This sort of terminology suggests that these people are not responsible for their actions, which are somehow beyond their own control; they were simply victims of their psychological lapse or environmental circumstances. These are examples of intermittent attribution. Yet individuals who actually *do* have a mental illness cannot escape that illness and must live with the ongoing victimization that results, internally and externally. As Sontag (1989) notes, "the metaphor implements the way particularly dreaded diseases are envisaged as an alien 'other,' the move from the demonization of the illness to the attribution of fault to the patient is an inevitable one, no matter if patients are thought of as victims. Victims suggest innocence. And innocence, by the inexorable logic that governs all relational terms, suggests guilt" (p. 99).

Sontag continues: "Illness is the night-side of life, a more onerous citizenship. Everyone who is born holds dual citizenship, in the kingdom of the well and in the kingdom of the sick" (1978, p. 3). She is not analyzing the process of moving to the place of the ill, or living in the place of the ill, but rather is challenging the ideas that society has of that place, and how metaphor is used to describe, stereotype, and stigmatize the "tribe" of the ill. She believes that true healing from stigmatization comes only when metaphors are excavated, deconstructed, and removed, so that the citizens of the "kingdom of the sick" have been emancipated to a place where they can be free of the "trappings of metaphor" (Sontag, 1978, 1989).

Youth and the Social Construction of Mental Illness

■ MENTAL ILLNESS is as much a social as a physiological condition (Illich, 1976). As one researcher points out, "for patients and health care professionals, it involves all the patterns of social life, interlocking social roles, power and conflict, social statuses, networks of family and friends, bureaucracies and organizations, social control, ideas of moral worth, aspects of work and occupations, definitions of reality, and the production of knowledge" (Brown, 1995, as cited in Lorber, 1997, p. 4). Lorber also describes the issues that affect how people are judged by and experience their illnesses (1997). For example, someone who has money, position, power, influence, a family endowed with socio-economic status, and so on, will experience mental illness differently than someone who has no societal status, money, education, or career opportunities (Brown, 1995, as cited in Lorber, 1997). They will be treated in different institutions, be prescribed different classes of drugs, have different disability plans, and have sometimes vastly different opportunities available to them in the community. Both will endure some stigma, but the person with a class or economic advantage will experience less obvious marginalization. It follows, then, that what people know about their illness and what they disclose to their network is socially determined as well (Lorber, 1997). For example, someone who has pneumonia and has to take time off work may be more likely to disclose the reason to his co-workers than if he is off work with a psychotic illness. Illnesses that are deemed socially acceptable are talked about, whereas those that are deemed unacceptable are not. If an unacceptable illness is made public, a person may experience various social consequences such as stigma and marginalization.

The social construction of illness also has a direct impact on how a person is treated medically or what "cure" is sought (Lorber, 1997). If a person has cancer of the throat or lungs and is actively using tobacco, the search for a cure will be influenced by how the physician and the patient view the disease and its root cause. That same root cause also has the potential to influence how research bodies respond to the identified problem and its etiology. Patients who are using harmful substances may experience "moral criticism or avoidance, both by professionals and laypeople" (Lorber, 1997). They may well be blamed for their illness and perceived as morally weak.

The patients may see it entirely differently, feeling that they are victims of their circumstances and that they have no control over the addiction; even so, they are left with guilt and are judged negatively for not being able to control their condition. In the same way, psychosis and other mental illnesses may be viewed as untreatable, as socially unacceptable, or as a sign of moral weakness; this places the blame on the individual. Like people with an addiction, those with mental illness have no control over their diagnosis, yet they are left with the guilt of having the illness itself and the resulting social judgment.

To understand the social construction of mental illness, we need to understand how people and social groups understand themselves or derive meaning. To understand the self in our society, we often look to images that are available in our culture (Lasch, 1979). In her study on photography, Sontag (1977) pointed out the importance of "self-surveillance" in relation to the images produced by the camera—that "reality" in contemporary society is increasingly produced by or through the photographic image. Our capacity to trust our own perceptions or decisions about what is desirable has been diminished. Images produced by mass media powerfully influence (Lasch, 1979; Sontag, 1977) how we understand and label what is "disapproved" (Becker, 1973) behaviour or "spoiled identity" (Goffman, 1963) in society. It is interesting to contemplate who might be the producers or creators of such images and how those images affect what we perceive as "normal." These images can affect what we aspire to as well as what we decide to comply with to meet social norms.

············

The Significance and Direction of This Work

■ EXPLORING AND DESCRIBING the phenomenon of mental illness as lived and experienced by transition-aged youth will help us understand the impact of mental illness on this age group. There has been little research on the subjective experiences of mental illness for youth that would illuminate how they live with their mental health problems, understand them, and achieve recovery. Young people have unique and personal knowledge of their own processes, from gaining an awareness of their emerging mental problems to their experiences of being formally diagnosed and treated. It is important to understand their attempts to make sense of their world, as well as their views of their ability to recover and to be future-oriented.

Information gathered from the life histories of youth experiencing mental illness may be useful for anticipating and identifying interventions that are more youth and mental illness specific, whether the interventions are formal or informal, program centred or system focused. These findings may help us develop policies tailored specifically for youth. The identified themes may also serve as a base for developing ways in which we can reach out to youth, and in which youth can reach out to help young people living with mental health issues live, learn, and work in an environment that is more accepting and supportive. Finally, the themes presented in this book may inspire researchers to engage youth in a particular way when developing youth-friendly programs; they may also sensitize practitioners to include the voices of youth when considering prescribing treatments and interventions.

....

Summary

■ OUR CURRENT UNDERSTANDING of young people's experiences of mental health problems is limited. The developmental tasks of late adolescence and early adulthood appear to be connected to young people's experiences of mental illness, in that the milestones of achieving independence, establishing a young adult identity, expressing sexuality, and developing a career contribute to the impacts of, and responses to, mental illness. The goal of relaying these stories is to open minds and hearts toward understanding that some people have struggles beyond their control. When this happens, we need to know how to be there, how to help them walk forward toward their futures with appropriate supports so they can succeed. People living with mental health problems do not deserve to suffer from stigma in addition to their internal factors. They need society's support. If this can occur, society will become a richer and more developed place and space.

To best plan for the developmental needs of transition-aged youth with mental health problems, supports and services should be based in part on the experiences and concerns of the youth involved (Macnaughton, 1997; McGorry, 1992; Ministry of Health, Ontario, 1993, 2000; Morrow & Chappell, 1999). Hearing and listening to youth participants examine, describe, and explain their experiences with mental illness may help other researchers and service providers better understand the experiences of transition-aged youth who have been diagnosed with mental health problems. These stories may contribute to a better understanding of the needs of transitional youth for service providers, policy-makers, and planners. Perhaps understanding these stories will also help community members, families, and educators to plan and implement supports and services that more effectively recognize and meet the needs of transition-aged youth with mental health problems. Finally, the results obtained from this research may help transition-aged youth experiencing mental health problems to articulate, understand, and relate to their own experiences.

TWO

How Do Youth Experience Mental Illness?

Carrie: *When you get sick, you are confused, so all your thoughts before about people and friends are—when you try to get back to normal and change your life and get new friends, it's very hard, because you are not looking at it the same way as you are not seeing things the same way … because you've changed, it's not the reality, it's not your reality, it's not your nature, so it's not the right way to deal with it now.*

THIS CHAPTER PROFILES how youth experience mental illness by outlining the prevalence of mental illness as well as the developmental tasks and societal potential associated with the transition from adolescence to adulthood. It also provides an overview of the relevant literature on transition-aged youth experiencing mental health problems from a developmental and identity focus. The chapter concludes by reviewing some of the problems identified in the literature for youth experiencing a mental health problem and by considering how gender differences play a role in these issues.

Prevalence of Mental Illness

■ THE CANADIAN MENTAL HEALTH ASSOCIATION states that 20% of all Canadians will personally experience a mental illness in their lifetime. Similarly, 10% to 20% of Canadian youth will experience a mental illness or disorder. An astounding 3.2 million Canadian youth aged 12 to 19 years will develop depression (Canadian Mental Health Association, n.d.). In addition, 70% of mental health problems and illnesses have their onset during child-hood or adolescence (Government of Canada, 2006). It is estimated that at any given time, at least 18% of children and youth in Ontario are experiencing a mental health problem and that two-thirds of this population have two or more disorders (Canadian Mental Health Association, 2000b). The rates of mental illness are similar for transition-aged youth. In May 2006, a Senate committee chaired by Senator Michael Kirby released a comprehensive report on mental health and mental illness in Canada called *Out of the Shadows: Report of the Senate Committee on Social Affairs, Science and Technology*. It concluded that "children and youth are at a significant disadvantage when compared to other demographic groups affected by mental illness, in that the failings of the mental health system affect them more acutely and severely" (Kirby & Keon, 2006).

The incidence of mental illness in adults and youth is similar in other countries. For example, in Australia, one in five Australians aged 18 to 99 experience a mental health problem, with 27% of younger adults aged 18 to 24 affected, compared to 18% of the general population (Brady, 1999). In the United States, it is estimated that about one in four Americans aged 18 and older suffer from a mental disorder (Kessler, Chiu, Demler, & Walters, 2005). Similarly, other research indicates that one in every four to five youth in the United States experience a mental disorder (Merikangas et al., 2010). It is estimated that approximately 20% of children and adolescents have a mental disorder with at least a mild functional impairment.[1] In addition,

---

1   Mild functional impairment is defined as anxiety disorders, mood disorders, disrup-tive disorders, and substance abuse disorders (U.S. Department of Health and Human Services, 1999).

children and adolescents experience severe emotional disturbance (SED) at a rate between 5% and 9%[2] (Merikangas et al., 2010).

A note of caution needs to be struck regarding data for rates of occurrence. Estimates of the rate of mental health problems may differ over time and from place to place because the definitions of mental health/illness change as a function of current cultural understandings of what is normal and abnormal. Also, age-related behaviour/problem behaviour is not consistently defined, described, or reported. Therefore, statistical reporting may not give an entirely accurate picture of the transitional youth population, meaning there could be false positive or false negative interpretations of data.

Some professionals believe that the onset of observable mental health problems largely occurs between the ages of 16 and 24. However, other research shows that 50% to 70% of all mental health disorders are present in childhood (under the age of 14) (Leavey, Flexhaug, & Ehman, 2008; Standing Senate Committee on Social Affairs, Science and Technology, 2006). In addition, initial research indicates that young people may have some sort of memory of identified mental discomfort at an early age. This suggests that there may be clues in what children know and say at very early ages that could help us understand they are struggling with an emerging mental health problem (Leavey, 2011).

Research indicates that the later the onset of mental illness, the better the prognosis is for individuals (Canadian Mental Health Association, 2000a; Malla & Norman, 1999; McGorry, 1992). This is attributed to older individuals having a longer period to gain life skills and academic skills before a major neurological or emotional disruption occurs. Research also suggests that early intervention and treatment for youth experiencing mental health problems results in positive effects in terms of physiological, mental, and social recovery, as well as in age-related developmental

---

2   SED is defined in children and adolescents as a "diagnosable mental health problem that severely disrupts their ability to function socially, academically, and emotionally. The term does not signify any particular diagnosis; rather, it is a legal term that triggers a host of mandated services to meet the needs of these children" (U.S. Department of Health and Human Services, 1999, p. 46).

achievement (Macnaughton, 1997, 1999; McGorry et al., 1996). Researchers in Australia emphasize the importance of early intervention in mental illness—in particular, psychosis—that focuses on the needs of young people and their families (McGorry, Killackey, & Yung, 2008). This early intervention entails reducing stigma, investing in evidence-based treatment, and empowering youth. In addition, mobilization, or youth empowerment, has been found to be vital to the well-being of youth as well as to their capacity to control the mental health resources they require to maintain their sense of well-being (Ungar & Teram, 2000). Early intervention also has the potential to minimize the "collateral damage" to social, education, and vocational functioning (Patel, Flisher, Hetrick, & McGorry, 2007).

....

Growing Up: Forming Identity and Developmental Tasks for Young People

■ YOUTH OFTEN EXPERIENCE stress, anxiety, and feelings of alienation as they transition from adolescence to young adulthood. Tilleczek and Ferguson (2007) warn of the risks for youth as they question their personal identity during these transitions. Social class, minority group status, gender, and cultural experiences all affect their ability to deal with the transition and can exacerbate mental health issues (Rudolph et al., 2001). In addition, students already experiencing emotional problems may suffer more than others during this transition. As one expert notes, "Depression, self-injury behavior, substance abuse, eating disorders, bipolar disorder, and schizophrenia have striking developmental patterns corresponding to transitions in early and late adolescence" (Masten, 2004, p. 310). Yet we know little about the impact of mental illness on the identities and developmental stages of transitional youth from this group's own perspective. This age group is of major importance given that, according to experts in first-episode psychosis, two-thirds of major mental illnesses emerge at this critical time in young people's lives.

Many factors influence mental health, mental illness, or a sense of well-being in youth. A youth's experience of a mental health problem has the potential to be life altering because the illness is likely to interfere with development and often delays or disrupts typical developmental milestones (McGorry et al., 1996). To make a successful transition into young adulthood, a number of developmental tasks must be accomplished, such as creating an adult identity, forming independence from the family of origin, developing relationships outside the family, accepting sole responsibility for decision making, choosing political and religious ideologies, and pursuing educational and vocational goals (Holmes, 1995; Stover & Hopkins, 1999; Wilson, 1995). Another key developmental task for transitional youth is establishing sexuality (Erikson, 1999; Stover & Hopkins, 1999). Even for the healthiest of youth, moving through these developmental changes can be challenging (Health Canada, 1997a, 1997b). Many youth with mental illness, because of the timing of its onset, experience a disruption in their high school careers and are behind in completing high school. As a consequence, the developmental tasks of achieving intimacy, independence, and so on are delayed. In addition, because this is an extremely important time in lifespan development, the social stigma arising from being labelled with mental illness is potentially damaging.

According to Marcia (1966), adolescents' ability to commit to a career direction and belief system helps them form their identity. He constructed four categories with which to evaluate an individual's identity status:

1. **Identity achievement:** After a crisis, in which the person has spent a great deal of effort actively searching for choices, she now expresses strong commitment.

2. **Foreclosure:** This person has made commitments but instead of undergoing an identity crisis, she has accepted other people's plans and accepts the role other people have assigned to her.

3. **Identity diffusion:** Uncommitted, this person actively avoids responsibility and may be aimless and without goals.

4. **Moratorium:** Though this person remains in crisis, she is on a path toward commitment and will likely achieve identity.

Marcia found that young people who fell into the first and last categories—identity achievement and moratorium—had the strongest sense of self. These individuals, then, had a stronger internal locus of control. By contrast, based on experimental studies, those individuals who fell into Marcia's categories of foreclosure and identity diffusion showed more variation in self-esteem. Marcia concluded that the harder a young person works to resolve his identity crisis, the stronger a sense of self he will acquire. These stages articulate the typical crises that adolescents and young adults are challenged with, but it assumes the individuals have the skills to move through the challenges based on "hard work." If an individual has a disability, the challenge can be greater and may disrupt the individual's progress permanently (McGorry et al., 1996).

In terms of Marcia's stages of psychological identity development, young people's sense of isolation, lack of milestone markers, and lack of ability to access work and education would predispose them to the stages of foreclosure, identity diffusion, and moratorium. In Marcia's stages, youth are in a state of crisis, unable to plan for themselves or to take on adult responsibilities. If this is the case with youth experiencing mental health problems, Marcia's stages could be useful when planning social and medical supports for this population (Schwab-Stone & Briggs-Gowan, 1998).

Meeting the developmental tasks of each stage is critical in forming a solid foundation for later adult mental health. Erik Erikson developed a psychosocial theory that holds that there is an "underlying blueprint for development that characterises all human personality growth" (Stover & Hopkins, 1999, p. 5). His theory outlines identity development throughout the lifespan with a focus on age- and stage-related developmental achievements—graduation, getting married, and so on. However, the psychosocial developmental hurdles encountered between birth and adulthood, and an individual's ability to overcome them after a mental health problem emerges, have largely been ignored by the mental health services system (Davis & Vander-Stoep, 1996; Vancouver/Richmond Health Board, 1998). Transition-aged youth with mental health problems have unique developmental needs as evidenced by the negative effect that mental illness has on young people's lives in the areas of family, friendship, career, intellectual functioning, and the ability to form and sustain intimate relationships.

The experiences of transition-aged youth who have been diagnosed with mental health problems have not been well-documented; as a consequence, there is no information about the needs of those youth as articulated *by* those youth. And the consequence of *that* is a mental health service system that is not as effective as it could be in delivering services to transitional youth, because of the dearth of research about medical and social needs based, in part, on youth's lived experiences. Historically, mental health supports and services have been planned for and funded based on observations provided by health care workers (Morrow & Chappell, 1999; Thames Valley District Health Council, 1997). Much of what does exist is published on websites or in policy documents, government reports, newsletters, and background papers, and it is often rooted in provider, political, or institutional perspectives. These documents provide information for planners and funders in order for them to build systems of health care and community supports to meet the needs of youth. In the past, services have not necessarily addressed the needs of consumers of mental health care. Consumers provided statements to that effect in an Ontario government consultation with mental health consumers, providers, and policy-makers that surveyed stakeholders' opinions on mental health service delivery (Ministry of Health, Ontario, 1993, 2000). While information gathered from service providers should not be discounted, the voices of transitional youth themselves need to be heard.

Defining Identity

We can define identity as the way people think of themselves in a variety of contexts: how they look and feel, how they achieve on the job, how they relate to members of their family and to other people, and what values and beliefs they hold and act by (Papalia & Olds, 1981). With the onset, and ensuing stigma, of mental illness, an individual's sense of identity or self becomes disrupted. Young people who are trying to become adults need to feel a sense of efficacy; they yearn to be effective, to do things competently, and to acquire a sense of mastery (Layton & Siegler, 1978, as cited in Papalia & Olds, 1981). Most people have some way to evaluate themselves in relation to the rest of society as well as a desire to measure their status (Goffman,

1963). Adolescents transition into young adult life by learning to relate to the community to which they belong and eventually integrating into society as productive and responsible independent selves (Erikson, 1963).

Self-evaluation is triggered by everyday events like looking in the mirror, having a birthday, and other "marker" events such as graduation, death, illness, and leaving home. People evaluate themselves in relation to the selves they know, in part by comparing themselves to other people (Goffman, 1974; Layton & Siegler, 1978, as cited in Papalia & Olds, 1981). Youth with mental illness may experience devastating losses in terms of social "markers"—for example, if they are unable to graduate from high school and are unable to leave home and live independently at this time. Layton and Siegler suggest that a crisis is most likely to occur if a person is unable to recover from a loss of efficacy. To apply this to mental illness, if a youth is unable to control her state of wellness over a protracted period, a psychosocial crisis is more likely to occur. A sense of self-esteem is difficult to restore or maintain once a person has lost a sense of identity and mastery/efficacy over her state of wellness or illness.

Erikson's developmental stages of identity versus role confusion and intimacy versus isolation form a context for understanding the transitional stage of moving from adolescence to young adulthood. Notwithstanding his developmental stages being perceived as gender blind, Erikson's stages of life cycle development and identity formation theory were valid and helpful in framing the theoretical analysis for this research. This context lays the foundation for understanding the typical developmental tasks that youth go through and the challenges those tasks impose. As a result, these stages provide insight into how difficult it can be for youth with mental illness to achieve those "typical" tasks.

Identity: Sociological and Psychosocial Perspectives

It is important to understand identity in the sociological sense. Since the 1950s, sociologists and psychiatrists have referred to identity as a self that is socially given and socially sustained. Identity is also recognized and governed by the roles an individual performs, by the "reference group" to which a person belongs (Lasch, 1984), or by the "deliberate management of presentation of self" (Goffman, 1967). Based on this theoretical understanding, if social identity and positive social adjustment refer to what is given and sustained by an individual's social group, then being isolated, marginalized, and stigmatized can have a direct and serious impact on a person's internal self-identity and social adjustment. This may to lead to self-alienation and self-hatred stemming from negative social feedback from the peer reference group (which in this case would be high school peers).

It might be that after the onset of mental illness, the social reference group becomes largely non-existent. These youth may feel great loss over separation from their scholastic peer groups. How does a person understand himself in such isolation, bereft of the access that his healthy counterparts have to work, sexual development, and typical social experiences? To achieve the goals of this transitional stage, individuals must possess a solid sense of who they are. Simply put, they need to form an age-appropriate sense of identity; they must have meaningful friends and relationships, the ability to work, and a sense of family; and they must feel integrated with others in the social community (Goffman, 1963; Lasch, 1984).

Identity: The Role of Work

Another important aspect of the maturation process is work. The role of worker is central to a person's social position and acceptance in society. The inequality of ability and capacity is such that the social rewards of work will differ (Hale, 1980). What is most important here is the developmental nature and context of work in the young person's life (Health Canada, 1999b). Given that young people with mental illness are preoccupied with surviving their illness, they may have lost their ability to achieve a balance of work and love. Therefore, a youth with a mental illness may be unable to achieve in the same way as a young person without mental illness, who has more psychosocial freedom to explore her identity through such roles as work, sexuality, and independent citizenship. Consequently, a youth with mental illness may well suffer from interruption of one of the most important social determinants of health: the ability to achieve economic stability.

Identity: The Role of Sexuality

The transition from adolescence to young adulthood involves the ability to move beyond identity crisis into a place of intimacy (Cohen & Hesselbart, 1993, as cited in Davis & Vander-Stoep, 1996). Identity and identity development involve many different factors. Sexuality often precedes the psychosocial transition into young adulthood. At this stage in their lives, youth are challenged to sexually mature, achieve a more mature self-identity, and find their place in society (Bettelheim, 1963). The physiological sexual maturation process in adolescence brings with it the initial psychosocial attempt at identity formation. This manifests itself as an almost complete preoccupation with personal appearance—for example, with "faddish attempts at adolescent subculture" (Erikson, 1968, p. 128). This concern with how one views oneself and is viewed by others is the first stage in the attempt at young adulthood (Health Canada, 1999b; Tipper, 1997). A youth who is unsure of his identity may avoid interpersonal intimacy. In addition, a youth who does not accomplish such "intimate relationships with others and with his own [sic] inner resources in late adolescence or early adulthood" (Erikson, 1968, pp. 135–36) may be at risk of being socially isolated.

....

Some Common Problems Experienced by Youth with Mental Illness

■ IN THIS SECTION, I review some of the common problems that youth with mental illness may experience and that may affect their ability to achieve the developmental tasks of this age group. Common problems include but are not limited to abuse, risk of suicide, substance use/misuse, depression and anxiety, homelessness, violence, and poverty. In addition, adolescent boys and girls often experience mental illness in different ways. It is important to note that similar research findings have been made in countries around the world.

Abuse

In 2008, just over 75,000 children and youth in Canada were victims of violence. Youth aged 15 to 17 report the highest rates of violence among all children and youth (Ogrodnik, 2008). One British Columbia self-report youth survey documented that 20% of female students and 13% of male students had experienced physical abuse. In the same report, 15% of female students and 3% of male students said they had been sexually abused (McCreary Centre Society, 1999). Statistics Canada indicates that sexual assault is the second most common type of violence committed against children that is reported to the police (Ogrodnik, 2008). Boys *and* girls are vulnerable to sexual abuse; however, 82% of victims are female. In addition, in Ontario, 62% of children enrolled with Children's Aid Societies showed signs of emotional disturbance and mental health problems where there were coexisting caregiver/parental problems (Canadian Mental Health Association, 2000a). Finally, a systematic review of evidence determined that there is an association between sexual abuse and diagnosis of mental illness (Chen et al., 2010).

In a study conducted at a large urban Canadian psychiatric facility, 83% of female adult psychiatric in-patients reported having experienced sexual or physical abuse as children or adults (Firsten, 1991). Similarly, in a US longitudinal study, data collected from 375 transition-aged youth showed that 80% of subjects who reported a history of physical and/or sexual abuse exhibited at least one psychiatric disorder at 21 years of age (Silverman, Reinherz, & Giaconia, 1996). In addition, a New Zealand longitudinal study showed that children exposed to sexual abuse were at increased risk of psychiatric problems and adjustment difficulties at age 18 (Lynskey & Fergusson, 1997).

Suicide

Some young people choose suicide as a way of coping with difficult circumstances. In Canada, suicide is the second leading cause of death among Canadian youth aged 15 to 24, after accidents (Statistics Canada, 2012). Although the rate of youth suicide in Canada has decreased over the past decade, rates are higher than in the United States, Australia, and the United Kingdom (Kutcher & Szumilas, 2008). In addition, suicide rates vary by region. In 2009, 3,890 Canadians committed suicide. Of those, 202 were youth aged 15 to 19 (Navaneelan, 2012). In the United States, suicide is the third leading cause of death in youth 15 to 24 years of age (Centers for Disease Control and Prevention, 2005).

Female youth are far more likely to attempt and think about suicide, whereas male youth are more likely to exhibit suicidal behaviour and to complete suicide (American Foundation for Suicide Prevention, 2000). In the survey-based data from one research project, 4% of males and 9% of females reported having attempted suicide (McCreary Centre Society, 1999). In addition, youth from low-income families are at a higher risk for suicide than those from higher-SES families (Cheung & Dewa, 2006). A questionnaire completed by Swedish and Turkish adolescents revealed that the following were significant predictors in youth attempting suicide: level of family support, pre-existing mental illness, lack of peer support, past suicide attempts, another family member's attempting suicide, and female gender (Eskin, 1995).

In a study examining the backgrounds of youth who died through successful suicide attempts, 42 of 60 individuals had shown signs of depression, and only 29 of those had been medically treated for it. The same study showed a high incidence of mental illness in other family members (Rich & Runeson, 1995). A Hong Kong study examined the deaths of 39 young people with the cause stated as successful suicide. Results showed that the youth experienced frustrating and disappointing events, internal conflict and depression, long-term family problems, and mental illness (Lau, 1994). Survey data of 108 adolescents showed significant correlation between family conflict, life stress, family and peers attempting suicide, and suicidal ideation and attempted or completed suicide (Ward, 1992).

Finally, there is a growing concern regarding the link between suicide risk and LGBTQ (lesbian, gay, bisexual, trans, two-spirit, queer, and questioning) youth. It has been widely reported that this population's risk may be two to three times greater, especially among male youth (ECHRT, 2013). Research indicates that 33% of LGBTQ youth have attempted suicide compared to 7% of youth in general.

Substance Use/Misuse

Canadian studies have indicated that the three most used drugs among youth are tobacco, alcohol, and cannabis (Vega et al., 2002). Males aged 15 to 19 are more likely to smoke than females (Health Canada, 2012). Research from Health Canada also showed a significant correlation between nicotine dependence and the use of marijuana in young people aged 15 to 24 years (2012). Another study indicated that use of cannabis among youth aged 15 to 24 was three times higher than among adults 25 and older, and that use of drugs such as cocaine, speed, hallucinogens, ecstasy, and heroin was five times higher (Health Canada, 2011). A review of major studies reported a correlation between mental disorders and substance use (including tobacco and alcohol) and determined that people with substance abuse issues had the highest rates of mental disorders (Jane-Llopis & Matytsina, 2006).

A Statistics Canada study indicated that youth aged 15 to 24 years were more likely to report mental health and substance use or abuse problems than any other age group (2003). The most common mental illnesses seen together with substance abuse among young people are conduct disorder (CD), oppositional defiant disorder (ODD), clinical depression, and post-traumatic stress disorder (PTSD) (Canadian Centre on Substance Abuse, 2013). According to one report, 25% to 50% of youth who abused drugs have been diagnosed with CD or ODD, while 20% to 30% have been diagnosed with depression and 16% with PTSD (Kilpatrick et al., 2000).

Depression and Anxiety

A British Columbia study stated that the most common mental illness among youth is anxiety disorders (Waddell & Shepherd, 2002). Another study indicated that 34% of students in Grades 7 to 12 report symptoms of depression, anxiety, or social dysfunction (Paglia-Boak et al., 2012). Research data indicate depression rates in children ranging by age from 2.7% to 7.8%, with the lifetime prevalence of depression for adolescents aged 15 to 18 at just under 8% (Cheung & Dewa, 2006). This research, based on Statistics Canada's Canadian Community Health Survey—Mental Health and Well-being 2003, also indicated that female youth have a higher rate of depression than males

(11% versus 4%) and that rates of depression are different for youth living in different regions of Canada. Similarly, a study of youth in Canada, Great Britain, and the United States indicated that female youth had significantly higher rates of depression in all three countries (Wade, Cairney, & Pevalin, 2002). In addition, this gender gap was evident by age 14. Other research supports the finding that anxiety disorders are more common in females (McLean, Asnaani, Litz, & Hofmann, 2011).

In an analysis of the Canadian National Population Health Survey (NPHS), researchers found that transition-age female youth experienced depression at a rate almost double that of male youth (Cairney, 1998). The NPHS also showed that adolescent girls aged 15 to 19 were the most likely to experience depression. Another Canadian study indicated that for both males and females, depression was most likely to occur between the ages of 18 and 19 (Health Canada, 1999b). Similarly, in a study of 89 youth in Jamaica aged 18 to 20, 36% of females had experienced anxiety and depression and 14% of males had experienced anxiety (Hilton, Osborn, & Serjent, 1997).

Homelessness/Street Youth

A Canadian Institute for Health Information report (2007) states that "people who are homeless are more likely to experience compromised mental health and mental illness" (p. 7). In a sample of Canadian cities, 12% to 67% of homeless people indicated they had a mental illness. Another organization, the National Learning Community on Youth Homelessness, found that about 40% of homeless youth state they have mental health issues (2013). In addition, homeless youth in Canada experience mental health problems at a rate of 2.5 to 5 times higher than the national average for youth.

The results of a face-to-face study with homeless youth aged 13 to 21 years in Seattle showed that participants came from unstable family backgrounds (a large number were from foster care) and that family members had substance abuse and legal problems (Cauce et al., 1998). Participants reported very high levels of emotional distress and mental illness, and almost half of the participants had attempted suicide. In a British study, homeless youth reported having experienced little affection while growing up, often with indifferent and violent caretakers (Craig & Hodson, 1998). Psychiatric disorders were present in 62% of the homeless participants. Results suggest that homeless youth experience high rates of childhood problems and mental health problems. In Los Angeles, the incidence of mental health and substance use problems occurs at a higher rate in the homeless youth population, compared to their housed counterparts (Unger, Anthony, Sciarappa, & Rogers, 1991; Unger, Kipke, Simon, Montgomery, & Johnson, 1997).

In one study, conduct disorder was the strongest theme among runaway and homeless youth (Booth & Zhang, 1997). In another study of 200 homeless youth interviewed in Manchester, England, 82% reported psychological symptoms and 43% had attempted suicide. Youth who were interviewed revealed that drugs were widely used as a form of stress management (Klee & Reid, 1998). Often youth see "the street" as the only alternative to intolerant, abusive, and dangerous home situations (Health Canada, 1997a, 1997b).

Violence

The media give much attention to youth and school-based violence. School-based violence ranges from bullying to verbal assault to the use of weapons, including knives and guns (Health Canada, 1997a, 1997b; Leavey et al., 2000; McCreary Centre Society, 1999). In a British Columbia survey, results showed that 50% of youth do not feel safe at school (McCreary Centre Society, 1999). Despite media attention to this issue, there is no particular evidence that the lives of youth attending elementary school or high school are becoming more violent. Research does show, however, that youth who behave violently at school tend to have a history of emotional and behavioural problems. Further, school violence and bullying experienced by younger adolescents has a negative impact on them as young adults (Fassler, 2000). A young person experiencing violence could potentially experience a diminished sense of self-confidence and ability to fully trust and relate to others. In addition, the stigma attached to mental illness can result in bullying by other students. A total of 21% of teachers reported that they had "very frequently or frequently seen a student being treated unfairly, bullied, or teased as a result of having a mental health problem" (Canadian Teachers' Federation, 2013). Further research is needed to explore the effects of school violence on the mental health of young people.

Poverty

In 2009, the rate of child and family poverty in Canada was 9.5%, a decrease of 50% since 1996 (Family Service Toronto, 2011). However, youth are more likely to be poor today than they were three decades ago due to high levels of unemployment (Citizens for Public Justice, 2012). Research shows strong links between poverty and poor health (Frankish, Hwang, & Quantz, 2005) and poor mental health (Capponi, 1997), and between poverty and poor mental health in developed countries (Freyers, Melzer, & Jenkins, 2003). Data show that the chances of youth experiencing violence and/or mental health problems increase by 50% if the family is poor. Thomas & Brunton's 1997 study showed that economically challenged youth 16 to 17 years of age drop out of school twice as frequently as their economically advantaged peers (as cited in Tipper, 1997). One study found that experiencing persistent poverty led to delays in children's cognitive, language, and socio-emotional growth, along with increased mental health problems later in life (McLeod & Shanahan, 1993; Dearing, 2008). These data have obvious implications for transition-age youth who are experiencing socio-economic difficulties.

Gender Differences

Research consistently reports that adolescent boys experience greater stress than do adolescent girls (Tipper, 1997). However, as children progress in age, the differential in males and females experiencing stress becomes almost indistinguishable (District Health Councils of Southwestern Ontario, 1996; Gove & Herb, 1974). Data suggest that pre-adolescent males show higher rates of mental illness than their female counterparts do. By late adolescence, male and female young people appear to experience the same levels of mental illness, and the proportion of individuals experiencing mental health problems shows a more equal distribution (District Health Councils of Southwestern Ontario, 1996), with the rate in females being slightly higher (Gove & Herb, 1974). A British Columbia survey of 26,000 youth established that 3% of male and 4% of female younger adolescents experienced emotional distress, rising to 6% of males and 11% of females in older adolescents (McCreary Centre Society, 1999). It is interesting to note that the types of mental health problems seem to have a gender differential: females tend to experience internalized disorders such as anxiety and depression, while males exhibit more externalized, acting-out types of problems, such as conduct and antisocial disorders (Offord et al., 1987).

....

Summary

■ THERE APPEARS TO BE a high incidence of youth mental health problems, yet there is a relative lack of research for this group from a developmental or age-related point of view. The research that is available for this age group suggests that the later the onset of mental illness, the better the prognosis, and that early intervention and treatment have positive effects on youth diagnosed with a mental illness. Working through the developmental milestones from adolescence to adulthood is a challenge for *all* youth. It is generally acknowledged that these transitions are difficult, even for the most typical or stable youth. Because these developmental issues can also affect basic mental health functioning, we can reasonably assume that the developmental tasks of social connection, work, educational achievement, independence from family, and establishing an intimate relationship will indeed be disrupted for young people with mental illness. Being diagnosed with a mental illness also seems to have a detrimental effect on youth identity development.

THREE

Youth Participants: Who Are They?

Alisa: *This is the first time anyone has asked me questions like this, and has been interested in my life further than symptoms and medications.*

I N THIS CHAPTER, I review the research objectives and goals. I explore why I chose a qualitative research methodology. I then describe the participants by profiling the 53 youth interviewed from Canada, the United States, and Australia. I end the chapter by providing a composite description of a male and female participant.

············

Research Objectives

■ MY GOALS AND OBJECTIVES in undertaking this research included the following:

- To help youth examine from their perspective how mental illness affects transition-aged youth on a day-to-day or practical basis.

- To elicit from participants their accounts and possible analyses of their histories and processes of becoming mentally ill.

- To encourage participants to consider and interpret the implications or effects of being labelled mentally ill on their social lives and on the illness itself.

- To have participants describe how their mental health history and its effects might relate to their psychosocial development and/or to the development of their identities.

- To elicit information on how the participants or others came to know that there was a problem, whether they had noticed changes in themselves or their environment in the past or the present, the effects of the diagnosis, and what they thought or felt about the assistance they had received.

- To provide input on the policy implications of the findings.

I encouraged participants to consider how their history of mental illness and its effects may have delayed the full development of their young adult identities, and how it may have interrupted the developmental task of moving from adolescence to young adulthood. Through their answers to a series of questions (see Appendix), most participants were able to reflect on and describe in detail their process of understanding the emergence of their mental illness. Most of the youth were able to integrate into their analyses an understanding of the mental health system on an individual basis in terms of being diagnosed and treated, as well as in the larger context of the mental health system. Moreover, most participants had discussed their problems and the mental health system with their peer group at the community youth mental health program they attended.

Essential issues that cut across all data were the experiences of being stigmatized and labelled (due to the diagnosis of a mental illness) and how these experiences may have interrupted the full achievement of developmental tasks, including identity development. These fundamental issues will be explored later so that we might more fully understand the experiences of these individuals. The participants' insight into their psychosocial development is a critical piece of this analysis.

Generally, I asked all participants questions about the relationship between mental illness and their lives. Responses sometimes differed between females and males, and not surprisingly, similarities emerged in same-sex responses. In general, females were more often concerned about being judged by peers and friends and losing social standing, whereas males were more concerned with family status. Both groups, however, seemed equally concerned with losing scholastic footing and vocational dreams and ability, although more females were currently working and concerned with future employment than males. Interestingly, the essence of what participants had to say was concordant despite the cultural diversity of the sample group. In fact, their norms, values, and interpretations of the social meaning of mental illness were similar, regardless of their gender or cultural background.

....

Why Use Qualitative Research?

■ THERE IS LITTLE RESEARCH AVAILABLE on the phenomenon of transition-aged youth experiencing mental illness. This research study was developed to specifically target youth with mental health problems transitioning from adolescence into young adulthood, and I used qualitative methods to elicit more accurate information from their own perspectives. As a result, I was able to explore and describe the lived experiences of transitional youth with mental illness. I was interested in how individuals and groups represent themselves through their lived experiences and how they create meaning from them.

I used open-ended questions to allow the participants to respond in their own words. I encouraged the participants to tell their own stories, at their own pace, and to disclose only what they were comfortable revealing. I made sure to establish an environment of trust and respect during the interviews, ensuring that the youth were comfortable sharing their stories.

A qualitative study asks questions that are "intentionally open-ended, so as to allow the member to use their own language and concepts in responding to them" (Emerson, Fretz, & Shaw, 1995, p. 114). The questions need to reflect relevance to age, stage, and topics that have meaning to the group. Ultimately, the questions in this study were developed to be closely related to the group's interests so as to facilitate the discovery of the voice of youth with mental illness, with the focus on the study's goal of under-standing the lived experiences of the young people themselves. The over-arching research question was developed to elicit information from youth themselves to address the present lack of information on the phenomenon of youth aged 17 to 24 experiencing mental illness (Leavey et al., 2000; McGorry, 1992, 1995; McGorry et al., 1996).

············

The Interviews

■ I CONDUCTED 53 INTERVIEWS with youth recruited from three differ-ent countries: Melbourne, Australia (25 interviews); Spokane, Washington (6 interviews); and Toronto, Canada (18 interviews and 4 repeat interviews). The three sites were convenience samples, as I knew them through prior research and/or clinical work. The interviews were conducted at community-based youth-centred mental health programs and a research centre, as well as in coffee shops. All of the participants attended community-based youth men-tal health programs located in large urban settings. I determined the sample size by recruiting and interviewing participants until no new themes emerged from the data. I recruited participants from three different countries to deter-mine whether different themes emerged as a function of location; they did not.

Because the interviewing process was based on qualitative methodol-ogy, I used an unstructured interview approach to enable the participants to describe their experiences in a deep, full, and meaningful way (Colaizzi, 1978; Glasser & Strauss, 1967; Osborne, 1990; Strauss & Corbin, 1998; van Manen, 1990). I conducted the interviews in a familiar, relaxed, and safe environ-ment so that the participants would feel comfortable in disclosing their experiences. I was attentive and available to each participant, achieving this by being aware of verbal and non-verbal behaviours and communication patterns. I used empathy, reflection, attending, and paraphrasing to facilitate the youth in telling their stories (Egan, 1998). The interview schedule (see Appendix) helped clarify, focus, and expand on points that were unclear during the interview process. Each interview was expected to last no longer than two hours. In fact, interview times ranged from 45 minutes to two hours.

....

Demographic Profile of Participants

■ THE PARTICIPANTS RANGED IN AGE from 17 to 26. The average age of participants at the time of the interviews was 19.75 (20 for females, 19 for males). The youngest age of onset of mental illness that a participant could remember was 6 years, in the case of a male who started having problems at that age. The oldest age of onset among the group was 18, for another male. At the time of the interviews, most participants were taking medications that helped them "keep stable and functioning" (Omar).

Table 1 shows the mental illness diagnoses of the participants by gender. Many of the participants had multiple diagnoses. For example, one male participant had received eight different diagnoses over a period of two years. The most frequent diagnoses were depression, psychosis, bipolar disorder, and schizophrenia. Male youth were more likely to be diagnosed with psychosis, schizophrenia, attention deficit disorder, gender identity disorder, and having a past history of substance use. Female youth were more likely to be diagnosed with depression, anxiety, a personality disorder, an eating disorder, a past history of sexual/physical abuse, and a past history of attempting suicide or suicidal ideation.

For the most part, at the time of interview, the participants saw themselves as very responsible about substance use. It was clear that the youth valued their mental stability and did not want to disturb it in any way. They were aware of the potential negative consequences of drug, alcohol, and "other substance" interactions. In fact, one male participant with a history of heavy marijuana use wanted to become an official volunteer to talk with other youth in high schools about the negative impacts of substance overuse.

Table 1

Diagnoses by Gender for Participants

Diagnosis	Male	Female	TOTAL
Depression	8	12	20
Psychosis	13	6	19
Bipolar disorder	8	7	15
Schizophrenia	7	3	10
Anxiety disorder	3	6	9
Personality disorders	2	7	9
Past suicide attempt/suicidal ideation	2	7	9
Post-traumatic stress syndrome	2	3	5
History of substance use	4	1	5
Obsessive-compulsive disorder	1	3	4
Eating disorder	—	2	2
Learning disabilities	1	1	2
Attention deficit disorder	2	—	2
History sexual/physical abuse	—	2	2
Physical problems (otitis media—male, hyperthyroidism—female)	1	1	2
Mood disorder	1	—	1
Asperger syndrome	1	—	1
Gender identity disorder	1	—	1
Seasonal affective disorder	1	—	1

I have created composite male and female sketches to provide an overview or summary of the participants. In addition, I have included a summary of my own reactions to the composites to provide a context for my experience of the group.

Composite Female Participant

The composite female was 20 years of age at the time of her interview for this study. The onset of her mental illness was at age 13. Her religious affiliation was Christian (mostly Catholic). There was some history of mental illness in the family, including schizophrenia and obsessive-compulsive tendencies. She did not have a history of using substances and was not using substances at the time of the interview.

Although she struggled to graduate from high school, at the time of the interview she was enrolled on a part-time basis in a job-training program at a community college. During her high school years, she had much difficulty socially and lost all of her friends due to the onset of mental illness. She sometimes had suicidal thoughts and much depression over the loss of functionality and friends in her life. She worried about her future and the fact that her dreams were no longer realistic, since her concentration and scholastic ability were no longer viable. She was angry at the illness for taking away the academic ability that she had enjoyed pre-illness.

The composite female was likely to have been assessed many times by her family physician and emergency hospital rooms and sent home with medication with little to no follow-up. It took many years for her to be properly diagnosed and prescribed the appropriate medication that relieved her symptoms. Because she experienced side effects from improperly prescribed medication, she strongly advocates that any person experiencing side effects from medication approach the prescribing doctor immediately with any complaints. She takes an anti-depressant and/or anti-psychotic on a regular basis and says that the faster young people can be accurately diagnosed and medicated, the less permanent intellectual and functional damage they will experience.

The composite female had experienced familial instability, for example, divorce and multiple relationships with stepparents, half-brothers, and half-sisters. This had caused her undue stress when trying to cope with her mental illness. Her social losses were probably the most devastating to her; they included the loss of her high school friends and people (including her family members) treating her "differently" once they found out she had a mental illness. For example, her friends referred to her as "weird," or her family assumed an overprotective stance. When her behaviour started to change with the onset of her illness, her friends completely abandoned her and she felt utterly alone. At the time of the research interview, however, she was working to make friends and establish a peer group at a program geared to serve young people with mental illness.

At the time of the interview, she was living either at home with her parents or in some sort of supportive housing arrangement. She was financially dependent on her family, for the most part, but was working part-time outside the home through a job-training program or was enrolled in a college training program to try to establish some sort of career. She was cognizant of her future and understood that she needed to work toward attaining a sense of independence and supporting herself financially.

Composite Male Participant

The composite male participant was 19 years of age at the time of the interview for this study. He was 13 years of age at the time of the onset of his mental illness. His religious background ranged from Christian to Hindu to Rastafarian. There was no known history of mental illness in his family. He had a history of experimenting with substances such as alcohol, marijuana, and Ritalin. At the time of the interview, the composite male participant was struggling to finish high school and was at a Grade 10 level. His scholastic career had been interrupted by the onset of mental illness, which had deleterious effects. For example, prior to the onset of his mental illness he had above-average or average marks and intellectual ability in school, but post-diagnosis his marks plummeted and his career hopes were dashed. He wanted to be an engineer, a doctor, or some other professional, but after the onset of his illness these intellectual possibilities were no longer available to him. At the time of the interview, he was a full-time adult high school student. He seemed over-dependent on family members for social interaction, approval, financial support, and recreational activities. Family life was fraught with problems such as multi-marriages, abandonment, violence, and immigration at a young age with difficult assimilation or integration.

Initially the composite male had difficulty getting a diagnosis. He was likely to have experienced multiple diagnoses, as well as some behaviour and conduct problems—for example, aggression and social appropriateness. He was admitted to an adult psychiatric ward in a general hospital and placed on medication. Accurate diagnosis, and the appropriate corresponding medication, took a protracted period to obtain. He takes antipsychotic medication on a regular basis and advises anyone with mental illness to get a diagnosis as soon as possible and get on the appropriate medication.

The male participants fit into one of two categories socially: either he was still enrolled in the public school system, was not part of the social mainstream, and reported being somewhat of a loner; or he had some friends prior to the onset of mental illness. But in both these scenarios, he experienced being completely abandoned by any friends he may have had and reported not having any peer support to help him through the onset of his mental illness. However, through attending a community-based psychosocial youth mental health program, he had established friendships and a peer group with others experiencing the same problems.

In terms of attitude, the composite male had at first been devastated by his intellectual loss and by the ensuing loss of future career prospects; but he now seemed somewhat philosophical, as well as hopeful that his future would eventually become acceptable, especially if he stayed on his medication and remained stable. At the time of the interview, he was living at home with his parents, attending a special education class, and being financially supported almost exclusively by his parents. For the most part, he was not focused on his future in terms of working toward financial or emotional independence.

My Impressions of Participants

■ AS A GROUP, the participants seemed somewhat delayed in their emotional and intellectual/functional development. For example, a 20-year-old expressed goals that seemed to be more at a 15- or 16-year-old developmental level. Perhaps this was because they had been disrupted in their role development at school, after being placed in hospital and removed from their peers. They seemed immature or delayed emotionally. For example, they did not appear to desire relationships or experiences outside their family home. Their ability to take even small risks seemed to be diminished due to fear of losing a sense of stability and having the facts of their mental illnesses exposed.

Most females were focused on trying to establish emotional relationships that their chronological female peers would have established at age 14 or 15. Female participants seemed to have advanced their academic/work careers further than their male counterparts. This seemed to be consistent with their ability to understand the need to work toward an independent adult identity. In contrast, at 20 years of age, males were still trying to finish high school with a self-reported limited intellectual ability. Males seemed even less advanced or mature emotionally than their female counterparts. They did not necessarily see the need for individuating from their families. They were still concerned with fitting in with their family of origin and being supported by them.

However, the participant group had an antithetical effect on me in terms of understanding their maturation processes. Because their circumstances put participants in the position of having to deal with devastating biopsychosocial challenges, this group impressed me in that they had learned to take a philosophical approach to living. They had learned to deal with the here and now and to live their lives one day at a time. They did not take anything for granted, especially their mental states or their understanding of reality. In this way the group seemed to possess a certain wisdom that was beyond their chronological years.

Summary

■ THE GOAL OF THIS RESEARCH was to have youth chronicle their stories and interpret (if possible) their process of becoming mentally ill. I used a qualitative research methodology to allow participants to discuss their problems and experiences with being diagnosed with mental illness and its effects on their development. The participants experienced a range of diagnoses, with depression, psychosis, bipolar disorder, and schizophrenia being the most common. The participants seemed delayed in terms of their emotional and intellectual/functional development, yet their ability to take a philosophical approach to living as a result of dealing with a mental illness diagnosis showed a maturity beyond what would be expected for their age group.

FOUR

Youth Speak:
Mental Health Experiences and Needs

Nadeene: *When I was first diagnosed with schizophrenia, my family didn't want to listen to me, they didn't know how [to act], I guess—they were angry, they treated me differently, like they didn't want to listen to me, and like they were [tuning] me out.*

THIS CHAPTER REVIEWS how I coded and analyzed the interview data and describes the dimensions that emerged. I portray the participants' experiences from their own perspectives, annotating their stories and making use of direct quotes. I focus on youth voicing their values and on how they create meaning and life direction while experiencing mental illness. The participants describe how they remember the emergence of their mental illness; their experiences and feelings around multiple social losses; their feelings of stigma, shame, marginalization, self-marginalization, and abject social isolation; and what it took to adapt and cope with the social illness and biological illness states. They also comment on the system of care in which they were involved.

Data Analysis: Emergence, Loss, Adaptation, and Recovery (ELAR)

■ I FIRST ANALYZED THE DATA using open coding. As I applied a constant comparison methodology, themes and categories emerged. Further analysis of the data revealed subthemes that could be viewed as *properties* and *dimensions*. Properties give the detail, and dimensions give the range or variation by which the properties or details of the categories can be understood (Strauss & Corbin, 1990, 1994, 1998). I validated the themes by checking with the original interviewees. I made sure not to filter or omit information because it might not have been an obvious "fit" with the themes, subthemes, and categories identified in the findings. After identifying the main categories, I read, reread, and coded the material to identify linkages between the categories as well as areas of overlap. The four main categories that emerged from the data were *emergence, loss, adaptation,* and *recovery.*

Emergence. This category represents how participants experienced their process of becoming mental ill as problematic. In particular, it covers how they experienced being labelled, stigmatized, and marginalized simply because they were now somehow different. Emergence includes the process of recognizing a mental health problem, being diagnosed, and possibly being misdiagnosed. Being labelled as mentally ill and the stigma of being diagnosed and labelled are also part of this category. It was the category most frequently raised by participants.

Loss. This category is about the process of losing one's sense of self or social identity. Participants at this stage experience a sense of multiple losses and arrested role development. Losses include but are not limited to the following: loss of identity, independence, family status, academic functioning, and social standing.

Adaptation. This category is about creating a new sense of meaning by adapting to the new reality of an illness identity. It involves learning bio-psycho-social coping skills—for example, accepting medication in order to maintain stability, learning to recognize symptoms and ask for help, and learning how to make positive changes in social relationships. At this stage, participants have started to gain a sense of stabilization, evidenced by an overall decrease in illness-related symptoms and improvement in overall ability to function. They have come to accept that they have a chronic problem called mental illness.

Recovery. This stage involves searching for a new self-definition and finding ways to ameliorate the problematized illness identity. Recovery involves re-emerging from the onset of mental illness and re-establishing social identity. The participants accomplished this by re-creating a sense of self in the face of the onset of a mental illness and the associated social construction and stigma. This stage includes regaining a sense of social integration and identifying strategies to maintain a state of recovery, including such things as locating the right therapist and being on the right medication.

Table 2 outlines the four categories, along with the themes and subthemes that emerged from the data analysis.

Table 2

Four Core Categories: Emergence, Loss, Adaptation, and Recovery—Themes and Subthemes

Category	Theme	Subtheme
1. Emergence	Emergence as problematic	Problem recognition
		Getting a diagnosis
		Confusion
		Lack of appropriate mental health services
	Multi-level disruption	Disruption in social and intellectual functioning
		Disruption in school attendance
		Disruption in cognitive ability
	Labelling	
	Stigma	
	Marginalization	Shame

continued

Table 2, continued

Category	Theme	Subtheme
2. Loss	Multiple losses	Loss of identity
		Loss of independence
		Loss of family status
		Loss of social standing
		Loss of being taken seriously
		Loss of income ability
	Arrested role development	Interrupted social development
		Interrupted sexual development
		Interrupted scholastic development
		Interrupted career development
3. Adaptation	Coping strategies	Medication
		Recognizes symptoms and asks for help
		Change in social relationships
	Stabilization	Decreased symptoms
		Overall improvement in activities of daily living
	Acceptance	Adjustment
4. Recovery	Re-establishing a social identity	
	Conditions for recovery	The right medication
		The right therapist
		A good doctor
		Family support
		Home-based treatment
		Positive attitude
		Hope for the future
		Community-based youth-centred program
	Reintegration	Volunteering

Overall, the essence of the interviewees' remarks was consistent. The four general categories or stages described above emerged clearly from all 53 participants. There were no significant differences between males and females or between participants from the three countries with regard to their experiences of emergence, loss, adaptation, and recovery. The youth experienced mental illness as a biological and social process for which they needed to develop strategies to recover.

....

What Do Youth Have to Say?

■ THE NEXT SECTIONS provide a detailed examination of the four categories, including quotes from the participants.

1. Emergence

Participants described becoming "mentally ill" as a process with stages. The emergence stage includes a number of aspects. The diagnosis of mental illness is often associated with a number of problems, such as problem recognition, getting a diagnosis, confusion, and lack of appropriate mental health services. The emergence stage also includes multi-level disruptions, such as disruption in social and intellectual functioning, disruption in school attendance, and disruption in cognitive ability. Youth in the emergence stage also experience labelling, stigma, and marginalization, including feelings of shame.

Emergence as Problematic

The youth indicated that as their mental illness emerged, it became problematic in a number of ways. The male participants experienced the onset of mental illness at various ages (between 6 and 18 years) and experienced multiple episodes of their disorders. Most often, they reported being admitted to hospital or another institutional setting:

Robert: *Like, I've done this many times, but this is the case that brought me into hospital, because I was very badly injured afterwards.*

Terrence: *For six months. Then I spent some time in the hospital, almost a month, and I was taken off the medication then. And after I was released from the hospital, I wasn't on medication.*

Female participants reported they were often sent home from the hospital or other institution with medication:

Seta: *They got a psychiatrist to talk to me, and he thought there might be a slight chance that I, that I am sick or something. So he diagnosed, he thought I was schizophrenic. And I took medication. Then after I got discharged from the hospital and I went back home and I went to see a psychiatrist, another psychiatrist, and I got—and from that moment on I took the medications and got diagnosed.*

The same participant described another occasion of being sent home from the hospital without getting the appropriate treatment:

Seta: *She would be very, she would think, "Gee, is there something wrong with her?" So what happened was that my mom and dad decided to take me to somewhere that, like the hospital or somewhere, to—you know, see what's going on, and when I then went to the hospital, I was acting very weird, saying—the colours on the walls were drab colours, and the doctors just sent me home.*

Similarly, another participant felt as though she was not admitted to hospital long enough to deal with her problem:

Naomi: *Or, like, don't admit someone to the hospital if you're only going to keep them in for two days and then have someone in that has a less severe problem and keep them in for a month.*

Some participants had multiple issues (e.g., eating disorders, unstable home lives, experienced racism), which suggests that young people had trouble with both biological and social stressors during the period of onset or emergence. The question becomes, what kinds of support are available to young people to help allay these difficulties?

Emergence as Problematic: Problem Recognition

The participants indicated that recognizing that there was a problem was often a process, though one that was not necessarily congruent with receiving an accurate or definitive diagnosis. This next participant stated that the problem had existed for a long time; the actual diagnosis came later through intervention by a parent in response to his self-harming behaviours:

Robert: *My parents were away for the weekend and so I tied myself up outside in the compost box and—really tightly, like so I had rope burns after this. And I just felt I wanted to be tortured. Can't really describe. Like this urge to be somewhere else, be someone else. And, well, I tied myself up and [pause] I eventually was able to untie myself ... I then covered myself in white paint. I just wanted to do it. No reason. And like, the idea of burying myself alive has been with me for a long time, and torturing myself. I'd get belts and whip myself until I bled. Just wanted to feel pain.*

Interviewer: *So you noticed that there was something wrong?*

Robert: *Yeah. For about 10 years.*

Interviewer: *Ten years. And then your parents noticed, obviously, when they got home from the cottage. So it sounds like both of you recognized at the same time that you needed to get some help, further help.*

Robert: *They observed that something was wrong with me, because I couldn't, I couldn't walk, my circulation had been cut off in my feet. So anyway, I was admitted to hospital the first time. I'd been doing this sort of stuff for years but it had never gotten this serious.*

Interviewer: *And so did your parents call, like an ambulance? How did you get to hospital? Or did they take you over?*

Robert: *They just took me.*

Another youth experienced a similar process. For a long time he felt something was wrong, and though it took a while, his mother finally realized he was suffering:

Sajith: *I think my mom did, and like—I think my dad just thought I was bad in school, but he didn't really think anything was wrong, but my mom, she like saw me more than dad, I think, and she knew that something was wrong and I was like 12, I think. Yeah. So. She was the first one.*
Interviewer: *So did she notice that you weren't very happy or—*
Sajith: *Yeah.*
Interviewer: *And did she approach you about it?*
Sajith: *Yeah, she just came up to me and touched me on my arm and she felt a big wound and stuff, and like she just freaked right out and I said yeah. That's when she found out.*
Interviewer: *A wound from where you were cutting yourself?*
Sajith: *Yeah, here. Yeah.*
Interviewer: *So she helped you then, she took you to the doctor?*
Sajith: *Yeah.*
Interviewer: *And the doctor referred you to a psychiatrist?*
Sajith: *Yeah.*
Interviewer: *You described to me earlier that you recognized you had a problem ... You knew since you were about eight—is that what you said before?*
Sajith: *Yeah. Like I'm not sure, but I think I had this feeling all my life, like I was always, like, aware that it was there, but I think I got more aware when I was like 10 or something, 8 or 10, I don't know.*

Another individual mentioned that his initial experience of having a mental health "problem" at a very young age (6 years) was negative in that the doctors gave no detailed explanation. A proper diagnosis did not come until he was an adolescent:

Omar: *Oh, like you see, when I kind of ... My doctor never mentions that time, that was [indiscernible] nobody put a diagnosis on me.*
Interviewer: *Did you have a diagnosis that you weren't aware of?*

Omar: *Well, being in this crisis house, but I mean, like, nobody ever told me that I was schizo-affective at that time. Nobody told me that. Nobody. Um. They did tell me there was something wrong with my thoughts, but they were not—they didn't know the official diagnosis.*

One male seemed to have had multiple diagnoses, starting at the age of 6 with his inability to speak until that age, and including attention deficit disorder, hearing problems, and a learning disability. This same youth was later diagnosed with bipolar affective disorder, obsessive-compulsive disorder, seasonal affective disorder, and borderline personality disorder:

Scott: *Well, the hard part is, I've been—I had problems ever since I was 6, like early stages, ever since I've been in school, learning disability and ADD and that, and I had a lot of things ever since I started.*

Emergence as Problematic: Getting a Diagnosis

Getting a diagnosis was part of the process of emergence, but rather than clarifying the problem, the diagnosis often exacerbated it. Most participants did not feel the diagnosis and/or subsequent treatment were helpful. They often used words such as "misunderstood," "confused," "saddened," and "hopeless" when describing their diagnosis, as the following quotes indicate:

Alisa: *When I was first diagnosed was when I was in the worst condition, I was like, not to say crazy, but I was pretty sick. My thoughts were confused ... I had thoughts that didn't make sense ... and I didn't know what to feel. I didn't know how to feel. I didn't know how I should have felt, how I was supposed to feel, because I'd never known anybody else.*

Terrance: *I think [being diagnosed] made me feel worse. Yeah, you know, sadder ... that I was able to realize what was wrong with me.*

Interviewer: *And now you're labelled and you feel even more hopeless? Because you have a label ... or ...*
Carrie: *Yeah, more hopeless because I have a label.*

Nadeene: *I wouldn't go to school, I would just stay at home, I wouldn't do anything, I was just really depressed.*

One participant experienced an initial psychological "relief" in getting a diagnosis, but it was not a literal relief. Instead, participants were relieved to know that somehow having a mental health problem was not their fault. In the longer term, however, this was not necessarily a relief from the effects:

Interviewer: *So are you saying that getting a diagnosis was helpful for you because people—believed you and you felt some relief. You knew what to do.*
Alisa: *After I went to that—you know, program at [hospital name], that we made it for sure, that you know, that I had a problem, I wasn't faking—you know, my mom was clear. I was really—I was relieved to hear that, my mom believed me that, you know, but I wasn't sure before about the shakes—whether I was gonna, you know, survive these things for much longer, because, you know, it's kind of like serious stuff.*

Emergence as Problematic: Confusion

Participants reported that their life was "normal" until a sudden plummet into "confusion and delusion":

Seta: *I asked the doctor when my illness is going to be over, when am I going to be back to myself? At that time I was very confused, because I didn't even know that I had a mental illness. I thought it was like any illness, so why does it take so long to heal?*

Alisa: *I had no idea why everything was going—was collapsing—not literally collapsing—you know what I mean. Why everything was going down the drain, at school, I had no idea—right until the doctor said something … I was playing my piano and the thoughts were coming and I suddenly realized there was something wrong with me, and the thoughts I was getting was—like they were interfering with my piano—not my piano, but with—with normal thinking. It bothered me, these thoughts.*

They interfered with what I was doing, especially with school sometimes. I was, in the beginning not making sense, my thoughts were not making sense and I was disorganized and like a person who had the weight of the world on my shoulders. My friends were always asking my best friend at the time—now that's at the time—"What's wrong with [name]?" and nobody knew what was wrong because I was dissolving in disorder.

Participants generally thought that their doctors did not initially know what was going on, so that it was difficult to get the proper diagnosis, understanding, and treatment. This difficulty led some participants, both males and females, to feel confused:

Zita: *My doctors didn't know what all was going on with me, because all I have, a lot of things together, for one year they didn't find what it was ... Yeah, I did know [what was going on] but it was kind of confusing to deal with it.*

Emergence as Problematic: Lack of Appropriate Mental Health Services

Most participants felt that they got help at the time they were diagnosed, but they were not sure it was the kind of support or help they needed. One participant remarked that no one asked her any questions to help her understand herself better (no talk therapy):

Alisa: *Mainly yeah, sometimes I feel like I'm not getting enough. Sometimes I feel like my psychiatrist is kind of lame, like, she's kinda boring, she doesn't say much to me. And I just—when I think of a psychiatrist I think of someone who questions me a lot, who's ... I don't know why, but when I think of a psychiatrist ... I think of someone very smart and like, quick and quick-witted.*

The same participant went on to say that the psychiatrist focused only on asking her about symptoms and medication, rather than helping her understand herself so that she could start to heal and regain a sense of identity or self:

FOUR

Alisa: *Like I want us to dig in my past and pull out the roots and pull out, pull out, you know, why—"Well, maybe you did this because of this when you were little, instead of this." You know, like those kinds—did you watch "Good Will Hunting"—like Robin Williams, like the psychiatrist, like that. That's how I imagine psychiatrists would be. That's who I wanted. But the psychiatrist I have currently ... focuses a lot on medication and the kind of medication I need.*

This seems representative of what most youth felt when interacting with their doctors. However, participants had a better view of their community workers and said they got a clearer sense of how to deal with their mental health problems when interacting with their caseworkers. One participant described how her social worker assisted her in her process and what therapeutic approaches helped her most:

Alisa: *Well, one social worker, asked me ... like they asked me these social worker questions. You know ... those questions that get you thinking, that you try not to do, try and impress people, I don't know. And they also—they'd given me a booklet, a white booklet, blank booklet, and they'd tell me to draw my family and draw things. That helped me express the way I'm feeling ... Like my social worker would say, "You know, why don't you hook up with Cindy? She's like you, she's like you," you know, stuff like that. Like they give you advice, they give you nice advice about yourself. That's what my social worker did for me. She'd even give me some one-on-one therapy alone, just me and her, because it was always with the family, it was family meetings we'd have, but in the end, when I couldn't see her any more, she did one-on-one therapy with me. And she'd say, you know, she'd draw a pie graph and she'd draw a second—sections, and there'd be one little section, she'd say, "This is OCD, but that's not all of you." Like she'd stress that "that's not all of you, that's only a little bit of who you are. You're also nice, you're also intelligent, you're also caring, you're also this, this, this and that." All these things put together. Like, that's an example, they did ... and they helped me understand, gave me perspective on what I have.*

66

When I asked participants directly whether going to hospital helped them, they tended to respond negatively; they saw it as unnecessary, scary, and disruptive:

> **Interviewer:** *And how was [the hospital] experience for you?*
> **Robert:** *It was a really bad experience. I met a lot of nice people but they had serious problems. And I felt really sorry for them, but like, I'd never cried so much in my entire life ... All they cared about was keeping people in line and—I never got restrained but I could have been if I had done anything.*

A female participant said that the hospital wasn't entirely negative, but the experience did not make her more hopeful or positively affected, and it took her away from her regular life routines:

> **Interviewer:** *And so what was it like in the hospital? You went to the hospital, you were there for a month and a half. How was that?*
> **Carrie:** *It was okay. It wasn't much, because I wasn't doing too much homework. It was like a time to ... time away from homework.*
> **Interviewer:** *So it gave you some time out from the real world.*
> **Carrie:** *Yeah.*
> **Interviewer:** *And by the time you were discharged, did you feel differently, did you feel more in control of your thoughts and a little more hopeful?*
> **Carrie:** *No.*

What participants clearly wanted from mental health services was for professionals to accept them and help them adapt to the change by assisting them in stabilizing. This could be achieved by examining a person's abilities and offering help in areas where they needed to develop more skills:

> **Interviewer:** *And in the mental health system is there something that's missing for people in general or for yourself, or something you can iden-tify? Or is it fine?*
> **Amin:** *Well, like ... the only part missing [in the mental health system] is, those people to accept who we are and, you know.*

Multi-level Disruption: Disruption in Social and Intellectual Functioning

Regardless of symptomatology or its degree of severity, a substantial number of participants reported an initial collapse of social and intellectual ability. For example, there were disruptions in ability to function intellectually at school and in social situations with friends and peers. These disruptions led to being stigmatized and labelled. Participants also reported difficulty in their roles as family member, high school student, and friend, which affected their identities. One male participant discussed the stress and disruption he experienced as a result of having a mental illness:

> **Scott:** *It was stressful ... Like, well, I had the real problems. I used to get in arguments with kids, you know, get into fights with my brothers and sister—my sister mainly. And argue with my mom and that.*

What is apparent from the data is that participants felt abandoned by family and friends when trying to cope with their newly acquired label of mental illness:

> **Alisa:** *Another issue I was dealing with when I was diagnosed, my social life hindered or deteriorated completely, 95%—well, felt like that anyways. 92 to 93% deteriorated ... My social worker, when I got ill, she came to the school ... She said that the high school I was going to posed a stress for me ... that it didn't help my situation at all ... and I was transferred immediately after that.*

> **Amin:** *First of all with my friends, like, I had many friends before I got my illness. After that I started to kind of losing them ...*

> **Zita:** *[It] was weird for me to faint, like—because people were talking about me in this high school, and that made me feel bad, and somebody—if somebody scream at me, I will fall down anyway, 'cause I cannot take it anymore. So it was like scary ... Yeah. I—in the school, people were just talking about me, they say, "Oh, look at her, she's just crazy, she's crazy, she fell down, she faint, she fell down that day," and this and that, you know.*

Carrie: *Yeah. And when I was went—when I went to school, I remember that I kept on laughing in the class, the whole time, and everybody was looking at me, like "What are you weird?"*

Sajith: *Because I was so depressed about school and stuff, I just didn't want to be there. Like yeah, people were making fun of me and stuff, and like, so it's just no place for me, it's stupid.*

Omar: *Well, my problem was—for me, like my main problem would be the shakes because I thought that, if I didn't have the shakes, I would be in school still. I would be, you know, I would be able to leave the school and go out and go on to college, right? So—but I didn't, I couldn't go on to college because my shakes, you know, it was like the main problem there.*

Alisa: *[Because of having mental health problems] I didn't do things normal teenagers did, like go to clubs, parties, drink, just stuff like that. Going out, I never did. I didn't do. I missed that part. So it was like I had a complete back—a complete gap between 14 and 19 years. Didn't really do things other teenagers did.*

The disruption in social and intellectual functioning experienced by the participants was quite evident. The quotes provided above make it clear that they were having great difficulty fitting in socially with their peers at school and with their families due to changes in their mental health status. Further, their descriptions of what happened with their peers at school suggest great difficulty in concentrating on schoolwork because they felt so alienated from the social world.

Multi-Level Disruption: Disruption in School Attendance

Many participants had to take significant time (one to three months) away from school when their mental illness emerged. In one case, a female youth was removed from the regular school stream at 13 years of age:

Seta: *Because I was sick when I was 13, I had to take some time off from school, because I was confused and not knowing where I was.*

Multi-Level Disruption: Disruption in Cognitive Ability

Disruption in cognitive ability, together with difficulty in concentrating, had a major impact on the participants' academic standing and their ability to maintain their studies at the same level as before the onset of their mental illness. Both males and females felt that their grades were negatively affected:

Alisa: *This illness, yeah. It interferes with my schoolwork and it's a really tough subject with me, because I—school is very vitally important to me, very important to me and I wanted to do school, but it's just—it's too much—like it's interfering too much—interfering and it's disturbing, because I used to do so well. Before I got ill I was doing so well.*

Seta: *Well, when I was 13, that's when I first was sick. And ... um ... I was doing homework in my room and the simplest questions I couldn't get. Like, I'm used to being a good student, I used to do very well in school. My mom and dad would be very concerned and would ask me, "Why don't you get this?" because it's just so easy. I was like, "I'm stuck, mom, my head can't think—my head feels heavy. I—it's not getting through to me."*

Labelling

Being labelled as mentally ill was problematic for many participants, as indicated by the following quotes:

Seta: *Difficult to accept that I am mentally ill. I felt very hurt in a way, that I felt really, really bad, like—I felt such tragic [sic] should happen to me, I felt like God had punished me or something.*

Carrie: *When the medicine and diagnosis is introduced, you start to believe that you're sick ... and you are not thinking of other things, of* *other ways to help you, you just think you're sick, you're—I'm sick, I'm sick, and you don't really know what's ... really wrong with you. I do not want others to know. I am cursed by god.*

The interviewed youth also reported having trouble accepting the label. One male participant expressed this difficulty as follows:

Interviewer: *And how did you feel about having that label?*
Amin: *Um. Just felt like, difficult to accept that I have a mental illness, but even though I can't but I have to, which is—I can't change it.*

Another individual described how it felt to be "different" and deal with the label of being "crazy," along with realizing that mental illness was a part of him:

Robert: *Had to face that I was sick. Or crazy. That was hard.*
Interviewer: *Can you describe what was hard, or define that?*
Robert: *Just realizing that I was different from other people. Like I always denied it, or wanted to deny it, but now I realized there was something wrong and it [mental illness] was a part of me.*

One participant described how cultural or societal images of mental illness affected her own self-image:

Alisa: *I just feel that I'm sad that I have a mental illness, because well, for one thing I'm just sad because I don't want something bad. I see mental illness as bad, a bad omen, and especially since society used mental illness as something crazy or disturbed people have. Like they have those TV movies where, you know, a person is compulsively doing this and they're thinking about spiders and spiders crawl on them. They make it so drastic, these illnesses, that people see it just as bad.*

It appears that a diagnostic label was useful for classifying the participants' problems, but the label was not positive for their psychosocial identities or self-esteem, as indicated by the following quote:

Seta: *I found out I had a mental illness and it shocked me like anything. And I was really upset. At first I was kind of angry. Not straightforward to God but just blaming, why it happened to me? And I didn't understand quite well why such a thing would happen to me, and so—I was mad at myself in one way.*

Since a person may lose independence and personal empowerment by being defined through a label, especially when that definition includes treatment requiring a hospital stay, it seems that most participants felt initially unsettled about the diagnosis and not immediately impressed with the treatment options. One female participant expressed the impact of being labelled as follows:

Carrie: *I didn't think that that was really good, because when—when you think of diagnosis, when you think that you have a sickness, so that you think that you are sick, so that's all what occupies your mind. So you don't really try, you won't see it as an advantage or maybe, 'cause you see that you're sick, and when you see that you're sick—you know that you're sick and you don't—you can't get better, 'cause you're sick.*

The following quote describes how one participant had internalized the images and metaphors reflected from society's stereotypical view of mental illness, and the effect this had had on her self-image:

Alisa: *Sometimes I don't like myself because, having to go through a mental illness is such a bad thing that I label myself and look down on myself. Like the way I see other people who have illness, like this is a very stereotypical view, but I think bad of others—like not to say to these people that I think that they're all bad because they have a mental illness, but just in general, when I think of mental, when I say the word "mental illness" it reminds me of bad, just bad in that—euw! Bad, who'd want that? You know what I mean? And I just look down on myself. But I realize my path through life has more obstacles than other people, but the light and the path, the light at the end of the path is more brighter—it has never been brighter or more visible than now, right? ... Diabetes is okay, but* *not mental illness. It's a very personal, personal problem. Nobody wants to know that you have a mental illness. Like no, what I'm saying, I don't want anybody to know I have a mental illness, because it's very personal, it means—'cause a lot of people think you're crazy or disturbed. It's a personal problem? So I don't want to advertise it [mental illness].*

Stigma

Participants had great difficulty in personally accepting the label of mental illness because of the stigma associated with it. The youth also commented on the negative change in social status after being diagnosed and labelled with a mental illness:

Alisa: *One more thing that really affected me, getting ill, was friends. I didn't have any friends. I don't know if it was because of the school I was in too, as well. The atmosphere was more—you know—everyone to themselves.*

In addition, more than half the participants felt they were treated "differently" once their friends and family found out they had a mental illness:

Amin: *And like, I found myself, that the group, they are treating me differently.*

Sajith: *Well—sometimes people treat me differently. Like I know my dad does kind of, and my mom, 'cause like—'cause like I can't—they can't fake, they can't really—I don't know, they just treat me kind of different. My mom—my mom knows there's something wrong with me.*

Some participants stated that their families treated them as though they were no longer capable of making "proper decisions" after being diagnosed with a mental illness:

Amin: *[My family is] not giving me enough independence, to be independent person ... but I have to tell them ... they can protect but not all the* *time, you know ... Like if I want the help I will ask them, but meanwhile I have to try to do my own, have to deal with my own problem, you know ...*

Strong feelings emerged about being labelled as "different." Participants stated that they now not only had a lifetime assignment of illness to cope with, but also the social stigma to bear:

Seta: *I sometimes think I'm so different from everybody, and I wish that I wasn't. I felt that, I wish I was a normal person. And I'd be so lucky if I could be this person or that person for a change. You know?*

A number of male and female participants felt that the social stigma and loss of academic standing were harder to face and deal with than the illness itself:

Alisa: *I had very few friends, and the friends that I had from elementary school that came with me to [school] I lost ... because I had a disorder. So it was very bad.*
Interviewer: *You lost them because they backed away from you?*
Alisa: *Yeah.*
Interviewer: *Do you think it was because they were afraid or didn't want to be associated with you?*
Alisa: *Yeah, or they didn't understand what was going on, they just thought that I was acting weird. Acting different. And you know, I probably was.*
Interviewer: *As withdrawn, you think? Is that what was happening?*
Alisa: *I was withdrawn, very quiet, my best friend kept telling me, you know, "Why are you so quiet?" And once, it was so mean, she once—she would, me and her were on the bus and she didn't talk to me at all, and I was like, "[Name], what's wrong?" And she's like, at the end, you know, before I left the bus, she said, "You know, I was treating you the way you treated me." Like I was giving her the silent treatment? I didn't even know that I was being quiet. I didn't know—you know how many millions of thoughts I was getting in my head, going all around my head? The anxious thoughts, the thoughts in general? Isn't that mean? Like, I think that's mean.*

Interviewer: *And she didn't know you were having difficulty?*

Alisa: *No, she had no idea. No one knew that I had a disorder.*

Interviewer: *So it seems to be something others have said, that their social life goes.*

Alisa: *Oh, definitely. Goes kaputz! You know, get close, splatters, collapses totally. Yeah. Like I don't want to even—it gives me a heartache to think about it.*

One youth comments on the image that peers had before an illness emerged:

Amelia: *Sometimes it [the mental illness] can change your whole mental process, the way your mind takes in things, because the disorder kicks in, and the type of disorder that I got, it changes. So that's why I think my friends would say, you know, "We want the old T back." Like one girl, she was my best friend from Grade 8 to Grade 9 and she thought—she's sort of getting angry that I wouldn't talk to her and she didn't know why, and it's 'cause I was creating—developing a disorder and as you develop the disorder, you know, you shut down, you don't talk—I didn't talk very much to her. I confide in her, be her friend, you know, but I was with her. And she would say like, "I want the old T back," and I would be like lost. I didn't know how she was meaning that. She didn't know that I was— I was getting ill.*

The danger of course is the internalization of spoiled identity, meaning internalized stigma. This adds to the already challenging state of having the physiological symptoms of psychosis and any other mental illness through increased stress, anxiety, and striving for social survival. One youth described experiencing internalized stigma as follows:

Liam: *You asked what is it like to have a mental illness? I think, it creates a lot of self-pity, feeling ashamed, look down on yourself. Even though— even though there's a hero inside, you know, it's hard to see that when it's obstructed by your mind's symptoms.*

Marginalization

Some participants felt misunderstood and marginalized and therefore "self-marginalized" in order to protect themselves. One female participant expressed her feelings of insecurity in this way:

> **Alisa:** *[I'm] so insecure about having friends. I'm scared that I'll lose friends all the time because I lost a few, those were very close friends … And I'm keeping a long-time relationship with friends in general, having commitments, being with friends. Having to meet them, because I don't meet them, I cancel because I'm so anxious, and they don't understand that.*

Females seemed more aware of negative social judgment associated with mental illness, whereas males were more concerned with negative family implications:

> **Alisa:** *Having the girls that were snobby at [school]. That was hard for me. I just don't like the fact that I lost a lot of friends, from the girls that came with me from elementary to [school]. They don't understand, they didn't understand, and I don't know if they would now either.*

> **Amin:** *Sometimes, sometimes [my family is] overprotective, but sometime you know, they, like I told them, "I need, I have to do this myself" … They say, "Okay." But the thing is … they don't just stay back. They will be watching me.*

Most participants indicated that they felt they knew something was wrong, but could not determine what was wrong and felt very isolated and marginalized. They did not feel there was a way to talk to their friends or families about their mental states. The following quotes describe their feeling of isolation:

> **Robert:** *I came back home and my parents wanted me to go to school and they eventually found out what happened.*
> **Interviewer:** *Did you tell them?*

Robert: *Um. I think they—no, I didn't tell them, no. They observed that something was wrong with me, because I couldn't—I couldn't walk, my circulation had been cut off in my feet. So anyway I was admitted to hospital the first time. I'd been doing this sort of stuff for years but it had never gotten this serious.*

Carrie: *Oh. I thought there was something wrong with me—because I knew there was something wrong, so I wanted to get out of it so badly, so I just told my mom, "I want to go to my doctor."*

The following quote expresses an overarching need for youth to learn to accept having a mental illness. Also, the concept of societal or social acceptance needs to be developed or changed to a more inclusive stance toward those individuals living with a mental illness:

Alisa: *Just trying to overcome the obstacle, like having an illness, accepting it in my mind, you know, I still haven't accepted it, I know, like it's very hard to accept something when you used to be okay and you used to be fine. You're normal, you know. Not to say what's normal ... you know what I mean. What's normal in society, you know. There's so many people that vary so differently in the way they act and behave and characteristics and stuff.*

Marginalization: Shame

Both male and female participants mentioned feeling ashamed of the diagnostic label of mental illness. For example, one participant reported feeling ashamed of his circumstances when his family came to the mental hospital to visit him:

John: *Honestly? It is like, it is time, okay—your family could bring stuff for you, you know, they were putting me things like fruit, vegetables, and all whatever, putting [it] in the fridge, I think. The staff in there would eat your stuff, they would eat, eat, eat, eat—like, I was on medication, medication there, but like, these people would line up for the medica-*

tion, people like—[grunting sound] and, you know? They're two seconds, sedated—tossed away ... I will be ashamed.

Another male participant expressed shame at being on disability allowance. He was unable to work due to his mental illness:

Scott: *I feel ashamed being on Disability. I do.*

Other participants complained that their friends and peer groups all but abandoned them once it was known they had a mental illness. One participant blamed herself for this:

Seta: *But then things didn't get better actually, things got worse 'cause I kept blaming myself for my illness.*

2. Loss

Participants described the losses they experienced as a result of being diagnosed with a mental illness in a multitude of ways. The multiple losses experienced included loss of identity, independence, family status, social standing, being taken seriously, and income-earning ability. The stage of loss also included arrested role development in terms of interrupted social, sexual, scholastic, and career development.

Multiple Losses: Loss of Identity

Loss of identity in the context of this research means that the effects of being labelled with a mental illness can cause a person to lose the typical process of being an adolescent and becoming a young adult. The following quotes show how youth cannot see themselves as independent of the illness:

Interviewer: *You said you felt bad about the diagnosis—did that affect your sense of self, your self-identity?*
Terrance: *Yeah, I was wondering what my purpose was.*

Interviewer: *How did mental illness affect your sense of identity?*
Amin: *[Identity] I wasn't aware of changing—So finally they got [an] answer for, how come—my personal change. I didn't know why—I mean, the doctor asking these kinds of questions, I didn't know anything was going wrong. So I mean, so—like finally my aunt took me to a restaurant, she told me that I got my [answer], which is a depression. So I said no way I have that.*

It is important to understand the sense of loss these young people felt when they either were diagnosed with a mental illness or experienced the physical and mental symptoms of being out of control. All of a sudden, they plummeted into a feeling or state entirely foreign to what they formerly knew. For example, one male participant felt very self-critical and self-depreciatory because of not being "normal" anymore:

Sajith: *I just don't like dealing with life. I just keep telling myself it sucks.*
Interviewer: *What would make it not suck?*
Sajith: *Well, if I didn't have this thing [mental illness]. Like, wrong with me … If I was just like a normal kid.*

The sense of knowing the self was gone. The safety of waking up and "knowing who you are," which most people take for granted, had suddenly vanished. One youth described the loss of a "normal life" as follows:

Robert: *Yeah, I was just, I was scared, I didn't want help, I thought I was the only person who had this sort of problem. I thought I'd never be able to live a normal life and—but then I learned there are others like me, and that makes me feel better.*

Multiple Losses: Loss of Independence

More than half of the participants indicated that they were still dependent on their families. One of the most significant effects of the illness for youth might be the continued or extended dependence on family for housing, financial support, and emotional support, given their age and stage and lack of optimism about their (future) independence:

> **Scott:** *But I always wanted to move back in, but I'm too old, I should be independent by now.*

> **Alisa:** *Oh, yeah. Ninety percent. I'm very dependent on my family. I don't like being away from them for more than two days. I depend on them for a lot, like, you know, to pay my ODSP, to tell them, I have to report how much I make from my café, to the ODSP, and my mom always has to remind me which, like, to get it into the government before a certain day, you know, like, your apron's downstairs, or you know, like reminders. Like, it's like she has two heads, one for herself and one for me, and I feel bad, because I know that shouldn't happen, shouldn't be that way. But I'm just more dependent.*

> **Amin:** *Yeah. Like they will watch what I'm doing, but then they try to go and if I make some kind of—when they know that I'm going to make some kind of mistake, then they just jump in. So like it's okay with me, you know, like—but the thing is I have to learn my own mistake, you know. But I'm trying so hard, which is—I don't know, I'm learning little by little. So everything's going so [indiscernible] that.*

Participants had a strong sense that opting not to take their medication had the potential to destabilize them and would be detrimental to their healing process. Therefore another level of potential dependence was pre-scribed chemical dependence. One participant described her world as scary when she didn't take the medication. She stated that whatever she did, she needed to remember to take her medication:

> **Naomi:** *Like, I said, "Well, I have generalized anxiety disorder, I have post-traumatic stress disorder, I am—like ... I have a mental illness. There's something I have that isn't right. [Therefore] I need to take medication for it."*
> **Interviewer:** *And do you have medication that helps you out?*

Naomi: *Mm-hm.*

Interviewer: *What do you take?*

Naomi: *Clenazapan [phonetic] 0.5 milligrams twice a day.*

Interviewer: *And does that keep you less anxious?*

Naomi: *Oh, yes.*

Interviewer: *And do you notice a big difference?*

Naomi: *Yeah, well, I've seen what it's like when I haven't taken it.*

Interviewer: *Yeah, what's the difference?*

Naomi: *I will ask the same question millions of times and I will have these racing [?] thoughts and it will take me longer to get my own tasks done, like hours. Well, 'cause one day—like, I think—in the night time I forgot to take it ... Yeah, well, now I just have to, like, remember taking [indiscernible] just whatever I do, remember to take it [medication], period, and then I won't have to go through that.*

Interviewer: *Yeah, 'cause then your body kind of goes up and down with emotion.*

Naomi: *It's scary, I don't want to see me like that.*

Interviewer: *Yeah, so you're like feeling stable and in control of your thoughts and things.*

Naomi: *Yeah.*

Multiple Losses: Loss of Family Status

As for mental illness and its effect on the family, both male and female participants found that their families treated them differently after they were diagnosed. In some cases, family and friends had all but abandoned them since they were diagnosed:

Naomi: *Well, when I was younger, my great-aunt, I—thought she was the coolest person ...*

Interviewer: *So does she not accept your mental health problem?*

Naomi: *Well, I said I have—she said, "Why are you going to the community-based youth mental health program and to the rehab training program? Like, what is the reason?" Because at that time I was in the transition period from the community-based youth mental health* *program to the rehab training centre. And I said, "Because I have a mental illness?" "You have a mental illness? You're not psychotic! Blah blah blah." And this whole big, like, debate on what a mental illness is. Like, I said, "Well, I have generalized anxiety disorder, I have post-traumatic stress disorder, I am—like, I'm mentally sick. Although I'm not like a psychopath, I still have a mental illness. There's something I have that isn't right. I need to take medication for it. It's mental illness."*

Interviewer: *She wasn't very positive.*

Naomi: *No, she—she very darkened [sic] it. And then—well, I called her in the summer, I called her that time in April, like, just before I turned 20, and then, maybe two months later I called her and—and she's like, like I'd call and she wouldn't be home, so I'd leave a message. And then finally, like one day I got speaking to her—and she's like—she said—she wasn't home when I called.*

Participants gave a number of examples of how families treated them differently after their diagnosis. For example, their families no longer appeared to trust their decision-making ability:

Nadeene: *When I was first diagnosed with schizophrenia, like, the change, like my family didn't want to listen to me, they treated me differently.*

In other cases, family members were more careful around them when needing to discuss a potentially difficult situation:

Amin: *Yeah, they pulling themselves away from me. So. Like, for example, like that, and then with my family, my aunt and some of my uncles, like my uncles used to be worry, strict and angry all the time. Like before I start to get sick. After I got sick, people were so nice, they never get angry at me, like they just laugh—now they just laugh [indiscernible] when there is something wrong, he just laughs.*

Participants also indicated that families were more worried about their whereabouts and happiness and were more overprotective:

Alisa: *[They] treat me differently since I got diagnosed with an illness. I think subconsciously, yeah. They don't realize it either, because they're overprotective. They want me home by a certain time.*

Seta: *I think my parents always loved me. I think nothing really changed except they worry more about me than before.*

Some participants described more tension in the home and increased fighting with and between parents and siblings. This conflict contributed to their feeling of being treated differently, which in turn negatively affected self-esteem and identity:

Scott: *Well, it affected my friendships—it didn't really affect my friendships, actually. It was really—my family members.*

Multiple Losses: Loss of Social Standing

Generally, the diagnosis of mental illness seemed to have had a negative effect (at least initially) on individuals' social standing. Loss of social standing refers to the external environment in which the individuals have no control over being abandoned in their social circumstances. One participant described what it had been like for him since his diagnosis of mental illness:

Amin: *Yeah, I notice that I changed a lot between friends and to—doing stuff together. But, the thing is now, like, I used to have like more than 30, 40 friends, like, I say now, I mean, they're involved with gangs and stuff, so—like I used to have many friends, now I have one, how many— two, three ... So I just kind of, like—not I'm more better, I'm different, you know. Like now I feel like a different person, but still like, I'm not that person that I used to be. I'm not as popular as I used to be.*

Some youth commented on a loss of social standing:

Seta: *It just—yeah, it's always a murmur in your ear, and it's whispering, and sometimes when I explain that to people, they kind of think* *it's very odd. Because not too many people hear voices and if you're one who hear voices, you feel like you're—queer, or like you're different from everybody and—and I guess those are some of the things that I would say were very hard for me at first.*

Interviewer: *Yeah. I can imagine.*

Seta: *Yeah.*

Interviewer: *And it's not something you share, as you point out, with all your friends.*

Seta: *Yeah, especially if you sit down with some of your friends who are, hey, you know what, I hear voices. [laughs] Weird! They all look at each other ... I see.*

Interviewer: *So the stigma of that is hard.*

Seta: *Yeah, the stigma is very hard.*

Multiple Losses: Loss of Being Taken Seriously Because of "Mental Problems"

Participants observed that in general, they felt they were not listened to or taken seriously when the mental illness emerged. This was evident in both the family and professional environments. One participant felt that he was having serious problems and was not being heard by the doctor or his mother:

> **Omar:** *The doctors in the hospital, they said I was faking ... My mother and brother thought I was faking it.*

One female spoke of feeling quite frightened and angry when she was brought to emergency because of suicidal ideation and was simply sent home. She felt that she was not taken seriously and consequently felt vulnerable being sent home during a time when she felt she was at serious risk. She spoke of increased anger and lack of trust in seeking help:

> **Naomi:** *The approach, being taken ... seriously. Like if you say, "I think I'm losing my mind," for people to take action right away as opposed to waiting until something worse happens. So the minute someone says "I feel like I'm losing my mind," get worried, it's okay if you feel you—*

there's a panic coming on, it's better that they [say] I'm taking this seriously, I'm checking you into a hospital, and even if at the hospital they say everything's fine, at least go to the hospital, and they could be able to do something. But the thing is, like, I've known people where ... they didn't take themselves seriously, or they did take themselves seriously, but the hospital didn't, and it didn't happen to me but it happened to friends, and I could have lost them, they could have died, because they had suicidal thoughts, and like ... have 80 pills, swallow 80 pills with water, and then would have to be hooked up to machines, and this happened and that happened, they drink tar ... so I'm saying, I'm not drinking tar, give it to me, I'll dump it out when they walk away. Then guess what, a week later, I'm back home, like, I know it didn't happen to me but what if it did?

Multiple Losses: Loss of Income Ability

Although only a few individuals mentioned economic struggles, the financial issues faced by this population require comment. Most participants interviewed in this research study were living with their parents or other relatives. Those who were not lived in a general state of subsistence, surviving on meagre government benefits augmented by part-time training allowances. In addition, for the most part the young people interviewed had not yet experienced having to be fully responsible for themselves, due simply to their age. One youth spoke of increased stress when socio-economic needs were not being met:

Amin: *Financial situation, like, it's hard for me to control everything in a tiny bit of money, so kind of hard for me to, you know, get—like I don't have enough support on that but I still have some kind of support, you know, a little bit of support from that, but not a lot.*

Another participant articulated his financial troubles, indicating that they were increasing his worry and stress level. He wanted to be independent of his family, but was unable to be financially self-reliant and therefore remained tied to them. He was not seen as, or able to feel like, an adult. The financial worry, he noted, did not help him in dealing well with his mental illness symptoms either:

> **Amin:** *My aunt, sometimes she advise me, too, but she—sometimes she helps me, you know, she say—if you need any money, tell me, I will send it. I said okay, I don't—if I need help, I will ask you. Even like, I think, two or three weeks, they had told me, like, "Hey ... do you need any—do you have any problem, do you want something from us?" And I said, "Okay, you know." And at that time I'm going through some kind of financial serious problem, and I asked, "Can I borrow this much money?" and she said, "Okay, come this time, I will be here. I will give you." And I went there and she gave me and, like, I think on this Saturday I'm going back over there, to my aunt house to pay them back, the money. So like they're helping us, but the thing is, I had to try to do myself everything, you know. Like they can help me, but not all the time, you know, because I have to try to do something my own. You see, I don't want any help. Like if I want the help I will ask them, but meanwhile I have to try to do my own, have to deal with my own problem, you know.*

Clearly, this individual was struggling with his developmental needs while negotiating the reality of the effects of his illness on his ability to work and achieve financial independence.

Arrested Role Development: Interrupted Social Development

In this section, I consider loss of social standing more from the point of view of what happens to individuals in their internal psychological worlds. A developmental interruption appears to occur when participants face the withdrawal of their social supports due to mental illness. This withdrawal has a subsequently negative effect on social identity and development.

Some participants experienced a high degree of ambivalence toward intimate relationships; they feared that people would focus on the illness instead of on them as young adults:

Seta: *I'm afraid of making friends because I'm afraid they'll find out that I have a diagnosed—and if I do have friends ... they're not close, though. They're just people from school that are in my class ... From the time I was diagnosed with an illness, I did want to make friends a lot, with a lot of people. Because I'm not sure what they think of me after they know the truth about me, that I have an illness. And it's also that, I don't know why, but I just don't feel like being close to people, like, being around people? I feel distant. I just want to be by myself, doing my own things.*

The participants also discussed how their diagnosis was disruptive because it caused social distance in their relationships:

Sajith: *When I was like, 17 or 16, I knew that I didn't want any friends and stuff ... I don't bother calling them and stuff. It gets pointless.*

Naomi: *No, but it's like—no matter how terr—how horrible people were to me in the past, I don't have to visit them, I can avoid—[indiscernible] like if there's tense—friction between people then—do not go anywhere where you're likely to see them.*

It seemed that females were more concerned with their social standing with their peers and described their social situations as more difficult since being diagnosed with a mental illness. Generally, those female participants spoke of being socially shy, finding it difficult to initiate conversation or show a sense of humour.

A few participants stated that, since being diagnosed and stabilized, they felt some social self-confidence returning, but it was hard to form "normal" age-appropriate relationships:

Carrie: *When you get sick, you are confused, so all your thoughts before about people and friends are—when you try to get back to normal and change your life and get new friends, it's very hard, because you are not looking at it the same way as you are not seeing things the same way ... because you've changed, it's not the reality, it's not your reality, it's not your nature, so it's not the right way to deal with it now.*

Although participants felt some sense of relief in knowing what was wrong, they indicated that it was hard to adjust to having a label and to having to start their social lives all over again. Females seemed to have less difficulty articulating the issues. They were more insightful about their roles and sense of social adaptability, although one female indicated that she had some difficulty taking on adult responsibilities:

> **Alisa:** *I was angry because I had to face the disease and my parents and brother didn't have one. "Why me?" Unable to behave maturely and accept responsibility during teenage years for my age, like to act my age, it was very hard. Like I was below the expectations of what people [think] of a 16-year-old.*

Some individuals said they had no friends prior to diagnosis, which suggests that disruptions in social development began before the awareness of a mental health problem:

> **Terrance:** *[long pause] Ah, well, even before I was diagnosed, I wasn't very outgoing, very social. And I wasn't as angry as other people, as I am now.*

In contrast, some participants found friends or a community through their diagnosis, which suggests the positive possibilities of organized mental health services:

> **Omar:** *Yeah, because [at the] community program, there's this guy ... and now I go to church with him. And I got some friends through him, right, and so his friends became my friends, and now I'm like—let's see—five other people from the Community Based Youth Mental Health Program.*

By joining a group whose members are experiencing similar social dilemmas, youth within that group do not feel deviant and can create their own norms and social opportunities:

Alisa: *Well, fortunately I'm part of a youth group, so there's about 20 of us and we're all friends, you know. We're not very close, we're good friends, we know that, you know, we're special to each other, like you know, we have that kind of relationship that we're in a youth group so we support each other, kind of thing. It's not just to plan activities for the next month, it's supporting each other as well.*

More than half of female participants lamented losing all of their peers and friends in high school and said they found that aspect of mental illness particularly devastating and isolating. Further, both females and males stated being abandoned by friends as a very significant and unhelpful feature of their process. Paradoxically, participants likely needed the support of friends the most at the onset of the illness.

Arrested Role Development: Interrupted Sexual Development

A majority of males and females stated they were not currently active or interested in being active in a sexual or romantic relationship:

Interviewer: *In terms of sexuality, do you ever think about dating or being with other people in an intimate way?*

Carrie: *I think—I think that's dropped a little bit. It dropped because it doesn't mean anything anymore.*

Robert: *I don't have any interest in females until I was 18. I was way behind. In other respects, too, but especially in that one.*

Generally, participants said they felt too emotionally vulnerable at this stage of their lives to be intimately involved with another:

Sajith: *Well, I don't think it's really ever going to happen. If I continue being fucked up, sorry, if I continue being screwed up, like, I'm not going to get one. Like if that—if that—'cause feeling stays with me my whole life, like I know I'm never going to get one. Like it's just inevitable.*

Alisa: *Yeah, I'm a little afraid. Yeah. So—I hear a lot about, you know, boyfriends, going out with your boyfriend and stuff. And I'm hesitant to go out with boys. Not so much fear of getting rejected, no. It's more, just how am I supposed to act? Like, what if they don't like—yeah, a little bit of what if they don't like me. So more just how do I act. Will they think I'm normal, will they suspect that I have something, will they, you know—I'm not going to tell them anything until, unless there's the one for me, you know what I mean.*

Other youth said they were interested in pursuing or "trying out" a romantic relationship sometime in the future, but that right now they had more "important" things to do, such as concentrating on finishing their education, establishing some career goals, and pursuing work/making a living:

John: *That's why I always keep an eye out upon these girls, because when girls—I don't know, like, they will play tricks from you, they will play tricks on you, they will do devious things to you, and they say they're doing it all in name of love. You know, it's like, nah. And I'll just keep a—I just like keep to myself.*
Interviewer: *So you think they're like toying with you or playing around with you?*
John: *Yeah. I used to take them home. I did it so that they wouldn't know what I'm thinking. You know, like—he's a very nice guy, but they don't know that I'm just doing it—like, I'm doing it to keep them out of business [indiscernible].*
Interviewer: *So now, no dating as yet, per se.*
John: *Um, yeah. Once or twice. But I mean, it was—um. There was a—let me see.*
Interviewer: *It sounds to me what you don't enjoy is—*
John: *Getting too close. Yeah. Yeah. Exactly.*
Interviewer: *That's too hard?*
John: *Yeah.*
Interviewer: *Emotionally?*
John: *I just leave them alone, you know, just leave them alone.*

Another participant described his feelings about dating, emphasizing the importance of studying:

Interviewer: *[Before the illness] you had lots of girlfriends?*
Amin: *Not a lot. But you know, like, I joke around with the girls, like I'm being in friendship with them and stuff like that. Now it seems people like—I told you about—you know, I'm not real interested in anything.*
Interviewer: *You aren't?*
Amin: *The thing is—before I used to like girls, but now like, oh, you know, as a friend, that's okay.*
Interviewer: *So take it or leave it?*
Amin: *Yeah, like now it's like—goal—I focus on studying and family problem, I don't focus on anything like that, I'm trying to focus everything I can and sometime, you know, it's doing like, oh, why should I see a girl? Why is she go me for [sic]? I don't even [want] her to go with me. You know. So like that.*

Some males and females reported having no desire or interest in being involved in a sexual relationship. Amin continued describing his views on sexual relationships:

Amin: *Before I used to like girls, but now like, oh, you know, as a friend, that's okay ... People I used to have no interest in, after I got sick. But now [it's] not 100%, it's around 2 to 5%.*

A diagnosis of mental illness affected the sexual identity development of most of the participants. One female participant expressed this as follows:

Alisa: *Since diagnosed I'm better able to handle a long-term relationship with girls or boys than I used to. Now I'm not saying I have boyfriends, I don't have boyfriends. But I'm—just in general, with girls and boys.*

Another example of developmental consequences of having a mental illness was this participant's social/sexual experience while living at a group home. A female participant described a situation she experienced with a fellow male resident and how she realized that getting intimately involved may have been counterproductive to the therapeutic milieu:

> **Seta:** *Well, when I was in one of the group homes, there wasn't any dating allowed or any relationships allowed, and what happened was I got into a relationship with a guy there, and it wasn't allowed, it was forbidden, and we didn't let anyone know about it, the staff or anyone know about it. And they found out anyways, and we got into trouble. Nothing bad. They just said, don't. You have to separate, you can't be together, you can't like each other anymore, stuff like that.*
>
> **Interviewer:** *How did that make you feel?*
>
> **Seta:** *I go, like, in my head, it was, you can't stop us. Like we have normal feelings [indiscernible], if we like each other, then we like each other, right? And then what happened was that we broke up, but staff said you guys are never going to be together alone, because—because it's the way he is and stuff, so. And we broke up. And I was pretty sad, depressed. And then nothing happened. Nothing else happened.*
>
> **Interviewer:** *Okay, was there anything that was unhelpful in your process that you can think of? Something that could have been better for you?*
>
> **Seta:** *I was saying that—I just wish I never had a relationship in a group home, it would be much better for me, because by having a relationship there it kind of—like, you know, we'd break up. We broke up, and—so people are taking sides of who to be friends with, I mean, it's hard—it's hard for staff too, because we both have our own staff that we like and stuff, so it's going to be harder. And I find that relationships and group homes don't work well, it's not a good thing.*

Arrested Role Development: Interrupted Scholastic Development

Participants clearly lamented the detrimental impact of their illness on their scholastic careers, wishing they could have done better and some wishing they could have continued in the schools that they had been attending pre-diagnosis (both high school and university students). The following quotes describe how some participants felt about having the development of their scholastic careers interrupted:

Robert: *Like, my goals used to be set really high, get high marks, go to university. Now it's just graduate high school and maybe go to college.*

Omar: *Yeah, I think I've become lazy with these career controls. These controls, I've now become lazy, you know, I can now prove to people around me, like, that I'm not lazy, that maybe I might look lazy only when I was actually sick and [un]able to do my schoolwork. Maybe that's when I was lazy, but now I control it, right, and they go—like, right back at you. I don't know if I have a diploma because nobody give me a diploma. I abruptly [indiscernible] Grade 12 advanced, so I guess I would get a diploma if I [indiscernible], because I get sick, I won't get the diploma. Like I [indiscernible]—what was you asking me?*

Scott: *Well, the hard part is, I've been—I had problems ever since I was six, like early stages, ever since I've been in school, learning disability and ADD.*

Some participants had previously attended private schools well known for their intellectual competition. Participants were very concerned that their scholastic careers had been interrupted and wished that their education had not been so adversely affected by a mental health diagnosis:

Alisa: *My grades, I had failing grades when I got ill. [I was] really quiet through high school, I wasn't confiding in my friends any more, I wasn't close to them anymore, and it might be useful for you to know ... before I got sick, I was very intelligent. Not to say I'm not now, but I was very smart and good with school, I had like straight A's ... It's a prestigious school, very, it's the most prestigious school in [the city], and I went there. See, that's the proof ... And that's the proof that I was smart, because I got in ... And that's what makes it all the more difficult to see that I have an illness now, because I was so smart and like, everything was going so well when it happened, and it really—I feel like killing myself, like, I feel* *like—euh! That everything had to go so bad when I was doing so well. It's like—you can feel the pain even more when you're doing well, before you got sick. My marks plummeted after two months of doing okay, like I was getting 78 and 77 in two courses, I was doing—averaging well—I was doing average to what other—I was on the average of what other people were getting, then I shut down from there. From there, yeah. And nobody knew why all this was suddenly happening to me. My thoughts clouded over my brain so I couldn't think clearly.*

Most participants were still struggling to finish high school, at an age when most without a mental illness would be in a university or college program, and/or be employed:

Amin: *I'm getting little, like good marks and stuff. But only problem is that attending to the school, but other than that I'm okay, and everything's doing so far good … First of all I have to finish my high school, anyway, so I have to get my diploma and stuff. And then I will be working on, which, you know, like, after that I can decide what I want to do.*

In addition, participants felt they had not recovered academically to their pre-illness state:

Seta: *Well, I would say that before I was—I was more alert and more—I was better at school. I'm feeling okay right now, but I was way better, way, way better. Like, during tests, when doing tests, I would be the first one finished all the time.*

Arrested Role Development: Interrupted Career Development

Many females and males were working, although the breakdown of the gender ratio varied per country. In terms of work goals, both females and males expressed a desire to work in the future. One male was interested in finishing his high school diploma and then going to trade school to learn a trade for a future career:

Scott: *In certain levels, I'm in Grade 12. Like, I can get—like Grade 12 in certain things. Certain things I'm probably Grade 11 or 10. My maximum grade is around 12.*
Interviewer: *Well, your goal is to get a skill—*
Scott: *Yeah. [Vocational] program. Get trained.*
Interviewer: *And is your worker helping you with that?*
Scott: *Yeah.*
Interviewer: *What kind of program do you want to get into?*
Scott: *Maybe—well, there's—a welder, a rob [phonetic] worker, something like that. You know? Yeah.*

However, some participants indicated that their career options were limited because of mental illness. For example, pre-illness, some participants had dreamed of becoming doctors:

Seta: *Yeah, I wanted to be a doctor, and it didn't work out because of my illness.*

Scott: *Be a perfect A student. Go to college. Be a doctor.*

One participant had high marks in school until the onset of his mental illness, which left him altered academically. He had wanted to be an engineer like his mother (and had the grades for it, pre-illness). At the time of the interview, he was 20 years of age and enrolled in a special education class, trying to obtain Grade 11 toward a secondary school diploma:

Omar: *Well, my main problem would be the shakes because I thought that if I didn't have the shakes, I would be in school still. I would be, you know, I would be able to leave the school and go out and go on to college, right? But I didn't, I couldn't go on to college because my shakes, you know, it was like the main problem there. Yeah, I was doing like, advanced, I was doing 81 per cent average ... math ... my favourite ... subject ... Yeah, 97% ... then I got diagnosed.*

In the end, participants seemed realistic and pragmatic about what career opportunities might or might not be available. They realized they had to lower their expectations and do something that matched their current level of intellectual functioning:

> **Seta:** *Yeah, I wanted to be a doctor, and it didn't work out because of my illness. And who cares, because I'm doing something right now that I enjoy doing actually. And that's what matters.*

3. Adaptation

The theme of adaptation includes coping strategies such as taking medication, recognizing symptoms and knowing when to ask for help, and changing social relationships; stabilization, including decreased symptoms and overall improvement in activities of daily living; and acceptance, including adjustment.

Coping Strategies

Adaptation is about creating a new sense of meaning through the process of coping. The *Merriam-Webster Dictionary* defines adaptation as "modification of an organism or its parts that makes it more fit for existence under the condition of its environment" (1999, p. 13). In every human experience, we learn to cope or adapt to our environments, whether the stimulus is experienced through the physical self, the emotional self, or the immediate or general environment. One participant described the coping strategies she used to adapt to her mental illness:

> **Alisa:** *And meeting friends at certain times, I'm better than I used to. Applying coping strategies discussed when in crisis, like, applying the coping strategies that I learned with my social worker when I got it, at [the hospital], … that was where I was diagnosed. And I'm better able to handle myself for when anxiety comes.*

Adaptation can be positive or negative based on a multitude of factors, including what environmental supports are available, what skills the person has, and what kinds of immediate resources are available (financial, housing, education, health, health care, and so on). How participants survived and perceived their process of adaptation is significant in understanding their healing process. Throughout the interviews, participants conveyed the sense that they had worked through great loss, confusion, and alienation, and had struggled hard to learn how to cope:

> **Amin:** *Like for example, I hated myself first and ... I hated what I do, and for example, like I hated my skin colour, I hated. So now I like, I've got back to—because for example, like, I know my friends love me who I am, what I am. So after that I'm loving myself, but first time, I hate myself, I hated doing everything, and I didn't want to even live. And I just felt like I want to end up my life ... But after, people telling me about my positive stuff, so I'm, now I'm back on track ... For example, now I don't feel suicidal or anything like that, because now I like what I'm doing, I know what I'm doing, so I love what I'm doing.*

Coping Strategies: Medication

Taking medication regularly emerged as a strong coping strategy. All participants were introduced to medication, and allowing for some adjustment (side effects, getting the correct medication, resisting medication), without exception, they believed the medication helped put their lives back on track. This, participants explained, was because the medication created a sense of stability. Most of the youth stated that medication was a critical factor in addressing their "disorganized thoughts":

> **Omar:** *The sooner on the medication, the faster the medication will help you and it'll help you right away and you'll stop getting the thoughts.*

> **Seta:** *I found that the medication before didn't work as well as the ones that now—because—the medications before makes me really tired and*

sleepy, and even though I eat a lot when I take the medication, voices—like, the reason why the doctor think I was schizophrenic is I told him I hear voices, and so—the voices don't go away, the previous medication, that was the first one. But this one, I take it and it's pretty good. Like I don't hear anything or see anything weird, unless I don't take it. If I don't take it, then it becomes worse for me. If you need it, then you take the medication because you know it's going to help you. It's going to stabilize you.

Scott: *I take the medication, which helps.*

In fact, all of the participants rated medication as the number one aspect of maintaining mental stability and a sense of control over the self, even if fundamentally they did not particularly like taking it:

Alisa: *Until I'm better. Until the medication takes effect. And they always say the medication takes four to six weeks, so that's why it's important to get them right away on medication, 'cause then they'll get better faster.*

Scott: *I was afraid about the Paxil part. Paxil was the first medication I took and I'm still on it. I was kind of nervous that I was going to die of the meds and I wanted to see if it wasn't poisonous ...*
Interviewer: *But you feel pretty stable—you're glad you're on the medication?*
Scott: *Some way yes, some way no. It makes you slow down, makes you tired, it makes you feel worse instead of better. What medication does for me, is—you're not hyper, it slows you down, you don't have the strength to do anything. You know, it's very hard. Medication makes you tired, gain weight, oh, it's very exhausting. Makes you have a bigger appetite.*

Interviewer: *And do you have medication that helps you out?*
Naomi: *Mm-hm.*
Interviewer: *And do you notice a big difference?*
Naomi: *Yeah, well, I've seen what it's like when I haven't taken it.*

Interviewer: *And would you say that staying on the medications would help me?*
Nadeene: *Yeah, oh, yes. Definitely. Staying on medication, yeah. Okay.*

Interviewer: *So you feel pretty stable on these meds.*
Omar: *Yeah. Yeah.*

Zita: *You have to take your pills, lately. Not because if you're not gonna—if you're not going to take it, you have to think yourself well. If something happen, just because I didn't take my pills, I'm not going to get better. If you do, then you're gonna—you're gonna see happiness in your whole life again.*

Coping Strategies: Recognizes Symptoms and Knows When to Ask for Help

Participants felt that another key coping strategy for adapting to the reality of having a mental health problem was being aware of symptoms and being able to ask for help:

Alisa: *I have to mature way faster to understand myself and how to help myself ... I know myself a lot more. I know that, and now it means that there is a time where you can get illnesses, mental illnesses, and like, you can get mental illnesses and there can be something wrong with you mentally.*

Participants stated they wanted to know as much about their mental health problems as possible and understand the strategies surrounding staying stable and how to "get better" or improve:

Carrie: *I want to know the way to get better ... And every day I try to see a way of how ... Every day I struggle how to get—how to getting [sic] better.*

Seta: *I would tell you that if you think there's something different about you than before, or if someone notices anything different about you, that you should go to a doctor, talk to him, he or she, and if he or she agrees that there might be a slight chance of something wrong, then do as the doctors say and go see a psychiatrist.*

Coping Strategies: Change in Social Relationships

After being diagnosed with a mental illness, participants described having to seek out entirely new friends because their former high school peers had distanced themselves. The youth felt a more stable sense of self-esteem if they did not pursue friends who had abandoned them:

> **Robert:** *Oh, I've made completely new friends. My old friends, I don't keep in touch with very much, because I deal with it, that's part of my past, and I don't really want to be part of it.*

Participants who said they were able to find friends or community post-diagnosis had joined a support group at the community youth mental health program (or one of its subsidiaries) that focused on youth-directed psycho-social support:

> **Naomi:** *And also what helped in [vocational program] was that people are all ages, and I can communicate with people my own age, but my talent is that I can communicate with people of any age. Because of what I have experienced in my life are things a lot of people do not experience, and that makes me able to understand anybody, and if they're—if they seem like a good—like an okay person, I'll talk to them, and that's my nature.*

More female than male participants felt connected to this support group because of the opportunity to establish friendships:

> **Naomi:** *Like when I left [school] I had maybe three friends, or—it's hard to say, I mean, I think I only left there with like two friends, or the one person—it became friendship later on, but I can say that—honest, honestly, I left—I definitely left with one friend, and that was it. But when I left the Community Based Youth Mental Health Program I left with like a lot more than one [friend].*

> **Alisa:** *And we're all friends, you know. We're not very close, we're good friends, we know that, you know, we're special to each other—like you*

know, we have that kind of relationship that we're in a youth group so we support each other, kind of thing.

Participants reported that their external support system helped improve family relations. The system gave them more of a sense of their own identities as young adults, rather than as a sick person or dependent child; the support group gave them a sense of independence. Overall, most of the youth seemed to be either working on or wanting to work on creating positive lasting relationships at every level. Some participants said they felt that creating and maintaining positive relationships was the key to success:

Alisa: *Stick to the friends you have and just open up to them and let them know, you know, this is something I'm going through and it's not normal, we know, and I know, and—just try and stick with them, and you know, pursue long-term relationships, because it's good to have friends, because you'll always need friends in the future, any time you need friends, to just open up to, to confide in, to share your tears, your laughter, your joy, your happiness, your emotions, you want to be—you want to be with someone, you want to have company, so stick with the friends you have. But if they're getting in the way, if they're treating you bad, change friends. Don't stay with them, change friends. You deserve friends.*

It is important and worth noting that the participants in Toronto were unusual in that they were all connected with a social support program in the community. At the time of the interviews, this was the only program offering these services in the Toronto area.

Stabilization

Some female participants stated that they felt more relaxed and positive about themselves since they had stabilized:

Seta: *The only issue I have now is keep on being positive. And keep on doing well, as I'm doing now.*

Interviewer: *Keeping yourself ...*
Seta: *Stabilized.*

Participants were asked to consider what issues they were facing since they became stabilized. One participant was very concerned about relapsing into symptoms and explained how she coped:

> **Naomi:** *Whatever I do, remember to take it [medication], period, and then I won't have to go through that.*
> **Interviewer:** *Yes, because then your body kind of goes up and down with emotion.*
> **Naomi:** *It's scary, I don't want to see me like that.*
> **Interviewer:** *So you're feeling stable and in control of your thoughts and things.*
> **Naomi:** *Yeah, and there are going to be days when—that I'm not fully myself even when I take it [medication].*

Stabilization: Decreased Symptoms

Participants tried to assess their current situation in relation to when they had first experienced the signs and symptoms of mental illness and were not as stable as they were at the time of the interviews. Most felt that their current situation was stable because they had a proper diagnosis and were on the correct medication:

> **John:** *I got a new medication and everything, and it's working good, you know? So everything's good. So okay, that's one thing taken care of ... I got my medication in order, got my education in order ... and everything, a job.*

Stabilization: Overall Improvement in Activities of Daily Living

The participants indicated that achieving a sense of stabilization improved many aspects of their daily lives. Some participants indicated that their concentration improved in school as a result of feeling stabilized:

> **Interviewer:** *Well, that's great. Do you feel better that you're able to learn differently?*
> **Scott:** *Able to do school now and that, yeah.*

> **Interviewer:** *Your grades went down and it was very hard to concentrate?*
> **Omar:** *Yeah, but when I can come back to schooling and go to college and get good marks—then I'll definitely—I came all the way back, you know.*

Others indicated that feeling stabilized helped improve their social interactions and family relationships, as shown by the following quote:

> **Amin:** *And maybe from the family I try to change, like I tell them I can do some things what I want, and tell them like not to be overprotective, and like give me a chance to do something that I want to do and let me try my own, without getting some help. And you know—some people they can learn from mistake, about everything they can to learn, you know. Sometime I have to learn by mistake, you know.*

Finally, feeling stabilized helped the youth in terms of their vocational possibilities:

> **Naomi:** *Present something, and then they will be impressed, and then they would say—well, I'm not thinking about what they wouldn't do, I'm saying, well, they sounded very friendly. I mean, I'm not going to say I'm going to start there tomorrow, because I mean, what I'm thinking is that I do that as a work placement.*
> **Interviewer:** *And get experience.*

Naomi: *Yeah, I mean, if I go there for a work placement a few months from now, then, like, that can be one of my placements, and another placement with the Body Shop and another place—I don't know exactly, but ...*

In general, the group felt that since becoming stabilized, they worried less and therefore could live their lives more effectively:

Naomi: *Worried thoughts, I do get critical thoughts; I'm able to easily snap out of that.*

They also indicated feeling more in control of their destinies:

Omar: *If I get successful, controlling myself, I mean, I think this would take me all the way, these controls, believe it or not, I believe they will definitely help me in school, and ... I think they'll definitely help me with everything, like I can definitely move on from this.*

Acceptance

Another common theme in terms of adaptation was learning how to accept the reality of having a mental illness. Further, participants felt it was important to start learning how to deal with that reality—in other words, learning to adapt by accepting a new part of themselves, accepting a new or altered identity, one that included having a mental illness:

Alisa: *Like I never thought of mental illness before I had my problem. I never thought that you could get a mental illness, and so now I know that I have to take care of myself mentally by taking my medication every day, by talking to a psychiatrist, to someone about your problem so that you feel better, so that you—people can solve them, help you solve them.*

This seemed to be the turning point in healing: accepting their challenge, adapting to that change in identity, and learning how to work from a new frame of reference:

Interviewer: *And your sense of self-identity, how has the mental illness affected your sense of self?*
Carrie: *Identity. I don't—I can't really settle on what I am because I'm always trying to get better and see things in a different way, things that are from reality, not from fantasy.*

This female participant also thought it was more positive to just be yourself:

Interviewer: *You're not as nice as before, meaning that you state your needs?*
Carrie: *Yeah. And I think that's why people accept me now.*

Participants seemed to feel that once they had the proper diagnosis and treatment, and realized that having a mental illness was not their fault, they could begin to accept and deal with what had happened to them. The youth were able to start distinguishing between the self and the illness. One participant aptly expressed this sentiment:

Naomi: *I own the illness, the illness does not own me.*

The quote below describes how a young person went through a process of getting ill, recovering, and moving on from being angry or disillusioned about losing her former view of herself to one of coping through a form of self-acceptance:

Alisa: *[After] about a year I showed signs of improvement, and I understood the problem, I thought, and I understood the problem I got wasn't my doing, it wasn't 'cause I did it myself. I didn't give it to myself. In fact there was no way I could have prevented it at all. And now that I'm 23 years old, I'm pretty much the old, I'm back to my old self—not completely as before I got sick, but pretty close. Like almost fully recovered.*

These quotes and insights from the participants show that recovery really has to do with believing in your own abilities despite having a mental illness.

Acceptance: Adjustment

After the onset of mental illness, participants had to alter their expectations because of the change in their overall ability to function:

> **Alisa:** *I'll never fulfil the expectations I had of myself before]indiscernible] one time, but not now. And I can never ask the same from myself.*

Some still felt a sense of loss around this but, for the most part, had accepted their new or changed state and wanted to move on with their lives:

> **Alisa:** *Not as angry in having an illness as I used to be, not as angry, like "Why me?" any more. I don't ask "Why me?" as much. I still do. But not as much.*

The ability to create a new sense of life meaning seemed to come from the process of adaptation or adjusting to the change in mental health status. This was achieved by adapting and learning new skills based on the new intellectual and emotional reality post-diagnosis to continue to respond effectively to the social environment. Participants had learned how to cope with the loss, confusion, and pain of alienation and were now oriented toward their future, a development that offered a sense of hope. One youth described this process of adaptation to or regaining of social norms:

> **Amin:** *Yeah. People don't recognize me when I have an illness out in the community any more, not like it used to be. I'm normal. I do normal functions, I go shopping, I have my own bank account, I visit my friends, I get along with people better.*

4. Recovery

The final theme, recovery, includes a number of factors, such as re-establishing a social identity; establishing the conditions for recovery, including the right medication and therapist, a good doctor, family support, home-based treatment, a positive attitude, hope for the future, and a community-based youth-centred program; and reintegration, including volunteering.

In their recovery processes, participants described re-emerging from their mental illnesses by (1) re-establishing their social self and (2) using strategic conditions that helped them maintain their recovery from their state of illness. Here is how one youth described how she was able to mitigate some of the negative effects of mental illness by controlling her attitude, or sense of self:

Alisa: *Keep believing in yourself, trying not to lose self-esteem, self-confidence.*

Recovery involves re-emerging from the onset of mental illness and re-establishing one's social identity. The participants accomplished this process through re-creating a new self-identity in relation to their mental illness. One young person described how her sense of self was altered because of her illness:

Alisa: *It was like my thoughts were critical of myself, deteriorating, not only my mental health but my self-esteem and confidence levels. I was not myself at all when I first developed the illness, I was totally out of character. Totally. No one knew what was going on, it was really strange, very strange. I had made very few friends while I—when I became sick and lost the friends I had.*

One participant described how she recognized she had a problem. She articulated her daily struggle to recover:

Carrie: *I felt that I know there's something wrong with me, there's something really wrong, and I have to fix it. And every day I try to see a way*

of how I can look at life a different way and get better, and every time—
every day I struggle how to get—how to getting [sic] better.

Another participant described how hard and long it was to recover from the onset of her illness:

Alisa: *My thoughts clouded over my brain so I couldn't think clearly.*
After two months of being on a mild tranquilizer, I stabilized. I was on
minor tranquilizer. And the social worker then at the time, at the same
time was sorting out my problems with my family and me. [After] about
a year I showed signs of improvement ...

Access to a community program that supported youth with mental health problems helped participants through the social recovery stage of mental illness. Having a community program geared toward social interaction and connection between youth with mental illness was a key factor in putting these youth in touch with one another. The program worked for the participants because it helped them develop a peer group where they could have a common understanding and non-judgmental view of one another:

Alisa: *So [talking with peers] helps me to deal with my illness better,*
and you know, suggestions they have for me, and I have suggestions for
them, that I give them on how to deal with your nerves and cope with
your anxiousness.

For the most part, the participants had a fairly optimistic outlook for themselves and their futures, largely influenced by the particular youth-centred community mental health program. The program offered youth a place to meet and form friendships:

Alisa: *I made tons of friends here at the community-based mental health*
program.

The program also allowed participants to access advocacy and case management services, employment training, and education:

Naomi: *Like I can always look back. Like the community-based mental health program is a place that will stand out, that they'll say, like, "Where did you make this?" I'll say, "Oh, I made this at the community-based mental health program, I did this at the community-based mental health program, I did therapy at the community-based mental health program, and I met these friends at the community-based mental health program and they're still here today." And if they ask me about the other places, I'll say, "Well, I didn't like it there," or they didn't know what they were talking about, they were clueless, but the community-based mental health program wasn't. I go to a full-time vocational program, I have plenty of friends, I never really feel lonely. I have music to listen to, I have written songs for people, a few stories, and mostly poems.*

The next quote describes a participant who was trying to set retraining goals. In the community program, young people are encouraged to set vocational goals by looking to the future through education and job training initiatives. They are partnered with multiple community work projects and community colleges that support young people with their goals:

Interviewer: *Do you have occupational goals at the moment? Are you working here toward any occupational goals?*
Carrie: *Well, what I want to pursue through the community-based mental health program is to maybe be a fashion designer, maybe.*

Youth said they enjoyed that the community mental health program offers youth a place on the program planning committee for input. This both empowered them and helped them develop decision-making abilities:

Nadeene: *Yeah. Well, there is a group [indiscernible] input committee here, where you voice your opinion and share your ideas and everything.*
Interviewer: *And you like that group?*
Nadeene: *Yeah, it's okay. It's like a— Yeah. It's like an advocacy.*
Interviewer: *So you guys can help direct the program?*
Nadeene: *Yeah, we advocate, yeah. We talk to people ... Yeah, this is a pretty good program, you make your own choices, your own decisions.*

Alisa: *I don't know if you know, but they cancelled the drop-in, and I wrote a petition to get it back [and the participant was successful in bring back the drop-in program].*

The participants also commented on the increase in their sense of self-worth since being involved with the community mental health program:

Nadeene: *I've opened up more since I've—when I was in the community-based mental health program … And I felt more independent, like I mean, 'cause I learned how to be more open. I learned how to succeed, I guess.*

Alisa: *Attend the drop-in. I love the drop-in. Then you know you feel like, normal. You feel normal because everybody else has a mental illness, and you feel part of a group and you feel loved, you feel unique and you feel special, you feel good here.*

In addition, having other youth with mental health problems with whom to talk and relate was meaningful and provided social support:

Alisa: *So having friends … to have friends to relate to who have mental illnesses as well, having the drop-in, the drop-in really helped me make friends here.*

Omar: *Yeah, because, like, at the community-based mental health program, there [indiscernible] was this guy who … and now I go to church with him. And I got some friends through him, right, and so his friends became my friends, and now I'm like—let's see—five other people from …*
Interviewer: *So all five of you go to the church group?*
Omar: *Yeah.*

Conditions for Recovery: The Right Medication

Some of the female and male participants said that being on and staying on the right medication was key in helping them remain stable. The following quotes demonstrate the importance they placed on taking the right medication:

Naomi: *[You] must remember to take medication that is right for you and speak up to get it changed if it is not.*

Seta: *But if let's say, there is something wrong with you and you need meds and stuff, then—then I think that the best choice for you is to listen to the psychiatrist and take the meds. But before you take the meds, ask if there is side effects to the medication and what's it for, and ask what is your diagnose [sic]. And don't be afraid to ask questions, because it's really important. It's always important 'cause you know for yourself what's going on. And so then, after knowing all that information, if you need it, then you take the medication because you know it's going to help you. It's going to stabilize you.*

Conditions for Recovery: The Right Therapist

Some of the female participants thought that having the right therapist who focused on a person's particular problems and helped them find solutions was very important to their self-esteem:

Alisa: *Oh, very good. I was close to my social worker. She gave me a lot of—she actually was more of a psychiatrist to me. She's the one that asked me, "Well, why do you think you do this?" or "Maybe you do this 'cause of this." She gave me a lot of coping strategies to deal with my anxiousness [sic], like she would like, tell me to list all the characteristics, good characteristics, what I like about myself and focus on those. Like what are the good characteristics I have.*
Interviewer: *So she'll challenge you.*
Alisa: *The qualities that I have. Yeah. And she did some one-on-one intense therapy as well, not therapy, counselling sort of thing.*

111

Interviewer: *So that helped, the one-on-one counselling.*
Alisa: *Yeah.*
Interviewer: *And your relationship, obviously—you respected her, and she respected you?*
Alisa: *Oh, yeah. Yeah. I got mad at her quite a bit but it was part of being close, I guess. You know.*

In contrast, other participants reported having had therapists who did not really "listen," which resulted in a lack of independent decision making. For example, some participants stated that doctors developed goals "for" them rather than allowing participants to decide on their own goals, as indicated by the following quote:

Alisa: *But the psychiatrist I have currently deals with, focuses a lot on medication and the kind of medication I need and ... and she also just ... talks to me, she also helps me with emotional feelings, the feelings I'm getting, you know, how I should think ... how she thinks, you know, I could be handling it better, emotionally. Just emotionally changing the way I think, changing the patterns of the way I think, to positive thinking ... I just want another psychiatrist basically.*

In fact, participants often found it a validating and empowering experience to tell their stories in a safe, non-judgmental environment during the interview process:

Alisa: *This is the first time anyone has asked me about my life; the psychiatrists only want to know about medication or my symptoms.*

Conditions for Recovery: A Good Family Doctor

Participants stated that to sustain a sense of recovery, it is necessary to have a good doctor who listens and accepts you for who you are. The participants indicated that the therapist's role was quite separate from the doctor's role: they expected to talk to the therapist in a non-hierarchical manner, and the doctor was there to be the expert on medication. However, they also expected doctors to listen to concerns about side-effects and to take the young person seriously:

> **John:** *Okay, my doctor, right, he asked me—so what the medication took me for—honest to God, I don't know. Some little tablets there with an X in them, and I don't know, guy. He said, well, I'm going to prescribe this for you. Like, I told him exactly what happened, right, all the mishaps and things. He like, he said okay, I can prescribe a better medication, and he gave me the rundown of the—this is a fairly new medication, it deals with chemical imbalances, this, that. If the doctor's willing to explain all of that to you, well, to me, I make up my—okay, he's doing something right. I can follow that. You know, as long as he brings it down to me, from my level, and I understand it, I will follow it. That is what I mean by a good doctor.*

> **Scott:** *Yeah, I trust my doctor, he's been in my family for 30 years.*
> **Interviewer:** *Okay, so you're saying that you like seeing your family physician because you like handling your own problems.*
> **Scott:** *Yeah. He's a really good doctor. I don't like seeing psychiatrists or psychologists because it makes me feel like a—that I have problems. And you know what bugs me? When people say, yeah, you have a illness [sic], it makes me feel like you have a disease? Or something like you're dying of something? It's not really like a disease or a illness, it's really like a chemical imbalance in your brain.*

Conditions for Recovery: Family Support

Almost all participants reported feeling as though they were treated differently after being diagnosed with a mental illness. Some families treated them as if they were mentally incapable of making a decision, that somehow the mental illness had permanently impaired their judgment. The following excerpt from an interview illustrates how families were unable to normalize the situation and behaved as though the family member was more his label than a member of the group:

Amin: *Yeah. And I don't like it, and I told them, I told my aunt when they talked about me and they said, like, I can't talk to you right in front of you because you will get upset or you might get bad[ly] influenced by that or [get] sad sometime, and so therefore we don't talk everything in front of you. So like, we're trying to help you by not talking right in front of you, and stuff like that. Then I said, "Okay, I understand."*

The participant not only had to deal with his family members not knowing how to act around him, and therefore, by default, disempowering him, but he also felt obliged to say he understood this behaviour. This put him in the place of the emotional caregiver for the family, while at the same time looking after his own mental health problems and dealing with the fallout of the label and the myths of mental illness.

Sometimes the general assumptions families made about participants when they were first diagnosed did change:

Amin: *Yeah. So [it] seems to me like they have more trust in me than when I got my illness. So they didn't have that much trust in me when I got my illness but now they kind of having lots of trust in me.*

This statement reveals that over time and continued experience with Amin, the family learned to trust him again. However, Amin also indicated that this process took at least two to three years. Therefore, it seems that what might have helped in this case was ensuring that the family members were well-educated and supported by the health care system as much as possible so that they could in turn offer support and guidance to the young person. Demystifying mental illness, supplying facts on mental capabilities, and focusing on ability helps families and young people by reducing fear and stigma.

This next individual outlined the importance of the family's role in early recognition of mental health problems. The scenario is telling in terms of what can be missed when families or society do not understand the signs and symptoms of mental illness, perhaps due to the lack of public health mental health education and the fear of stigma. The youth indicated that he had engaged in self-harming behaviours while his parents were away for the weekend. A few days after the parents arrived home, they discovered what he had done and took him to the hospital emergency room for assessment. He was subsequently admitted to the in-patient ward, where he felt misunderstood:

> **Interviewer:** *And so did your parents call an ambulance? How did you get to hospital? Or did they take you over?*
> **Robert:** *They just took me … It was a really bad experience. I met a lot of nice people but they had serious problems.*
> **Interviewer:** *And were you scared at all? Frightened in any way?*
> **Robert:** *I'm scared of doing it [self-harming behaviours] again. I wasn't scared of the hospital.*
> **Interviewer:** *So [was] the hospital there for you?*
> **Robert:** *The hospital wasn't there for me.*
> **Interviewer:** *No?*
> **Robert:** *All they cared about was keeping people in line and—I never got restrained but I could have been if I had done anything.*

This excerpt outlines issues that helped and that did not help in the process of accessing support for mental problems. Aside from the reason for this participant needing help, the experience was similar to that of other participants. It is essential that parents and communities understand the signs and symptoms of mental illness to facilitate early recognition and intervention.

Some of the participants expressed the importance of having a supportive family that accepted, loved, and attempted to understand them:

> **Alisa:** *Oh, yeah, immensely. You know, it's been wonderful, my parents support me—like all they did when they learned about my—that I had this illness, was read up on it. They read tons of books. They know more about it than I do, and I have the disorder. So I'm just very lucky to have such supportive family, and my brother—my brother did a research project on OCD and how it affects the family. And it was very good, very good report. And when they asked him, "Why did you pick this topic?" he said*

"My sister has it, in the family, and I want to learn more about it and I want to help her."

Omar: *Because my mom, she's the one who actually has faith in me, faith, and what I do.*

In contrast, one participant described what it was like for him not to have a family who offered their support:

John: *'Cause like when my father threw me out, oh ... I used to cry every night. Got workers [indiscernible] will tell you, when I first came to the house, I cried [all the time].*

It seems by the comments and experiences described by the participants that family support can play a critical role in their processes, if, of course, support is available and accessible, and the parents are willing to give it.

Conditions for Recovery: Home-Based Treatment

Most participants who experienced a hospital stay or time in a group home said that it was not necessarily a positive experience. They felt it might have been better if they could have stayed at home and received treatment in the community:

Interviewer: *What was stressful about living in a group home in particular, do you remember?*
Scott: *Like I— Just a few months later I go that there group home. It was hard to see my mom, I've seen her every weekend, and it was hard, I saw her less and less, and finally every—I hadn't seen my mom in two years when I, once I moved to ... Oh my God. 'Cause of my behaviour at home. You know. Oh, man. It was very stressful.*

The next quote refers to living in a training centre and what happened when the interviewee was treated badly:

Scott: *Two bad things happened to me there [referring to incidents involving staff and other residents]. That's why I started to hate group homes and that, you get more aggressive, you know?*

Another participant had lived at a group home since an early age. She described contact with her parents as unsatisfactory. She did not hear from them for two years. At the time of the interview, she was 17 years of age and had been living in an institution since she was 14. It is easy to imagine her loneliness and understand that living in an institutional setting is not optimal:

Naomi: *Well, because I was told from my social worker, or from the worker at the house, that I was—I was told, call after 6 because they eat dinner at 5, or something like that. So, okay, like around 6 or 6:30. So then the next day we did that and then we were told, or next week, or sometime, or—then there was a message which told, like, "Don't call him, he'll call you." And it never happened. I had these very angry feelings towards him, I was thinking, "What's up with this? Two years and he hasn't called."*

Another participant appreciated living back home with her parents, where she felt she had more privacy:

Seta: *I used to live in two group homes and then—now I live with my parents. I've been living with my parents almost a year or two, so ...*
Interviewer: *[What] do you like?*
Seta: *Yeah, because—like, everyone is in the same place, like you share everything, everybody shares ideas and stuff, and everybody knows everything about everybody. And sometimes it's not good.*

Some participants who spent time in hospital described how they felt about their experiences:

Interviewer: *What kinds of issues did you have to face ... You mentioned going to the hospital.*

Sajith: *Yeah, I had to go to the hospital and you mean, what kind of issues at the hospital?*
Interviewer: *Was it hard to go to the hospital. Was it frightening?*
Sajith: *I was pretty—Like at first like I was like—'cause I thought that the hospital was like totally different. I thought they would lock you up in a dark cell and like throw away the key and just give you stuff to eat through the—through a [sic] opening in the door and stuff. But I had no idea of what I was in for. Like—but [indiscernible—low voice]—*
Interviewer: *And so was it better than you thought then?*
Sajith: *No, it was just shitty … [indiscernible]*
Interviewer: *Shitty, did you say?*
Sajith: *Yeah.*
Interviewer: *Why? Because nobody understood you or …?*
Sajith: *No, 'cause like, I don't know, 'cause in the hospital it's like—it was really boring and stuff, and like aside from that I had these big, like beefy guys, they bossed me around and stuff.*

It appears that if young people could be treated in a community environment while living at home with their parents in a supportive environment, it would be less stressful and might accelerate the recovery process.

Conditions for Recovery: Positive Attitude

When participants felt they were recovered enough to look toward the future, they became more willing to build on their strengths. One youth stated that he was working hard to build a positive attitude for his future:

John: *You gotta work for it, so as long as it takes, you know? I got the time, to that degree, you know? … If I don't be positive, nobody can be positive for me, I think.*

In addition, in offering advice to other youth, most participants felt they must remain positive to have a stable and healthy life:

Interviewer: *If I were a young person and I'd just been diagnosed with a mental health problem and I was trying to get help, and you were here, and you're my peer, and I asked you for advice, what would you tell me?*
Carrie: *Just don't look at anything bad, just keep on going, keep your high hopes and just keep on going and just don't look around people around you ... or don't look at them or their habits, because—just do what you think you have to do and don't get caught up. [pause] Don't think of anything negative too much. Just keep on going with the good— because negative affects your thinking, if you think negative you're going to get more negative, more negative.*

Robert: *Accept yourself. Still a person, you can do whatever you want, it doesn't matter what mental illness you have or—let your life, you can still do it.*

Conditions for Recovery: Hope for the Future

Participants felt that a sense of hope for the future was important, all the while not dwelling on the past or on the social and intellectual losses sustained through the process of becoming ill:

Naomi: *I would say that life goes on. That anything can happen, so, um. We cannot be smashed, we cannot be defeated. Um. There's always something in a person that will make them want to triumph, no matter what happens, and that there is some source of life, there is some angel, there is some power grown out of all the turmoil and all the negatives and all the lies, there's always a path leading to [indiscernible] to news [?] and truth. That's about it.*
Interviewer: *You're very positive in your approach.*
Naomi: *Thank you. There's always that, in the end. And life is—like, just knowing that yesterday, like, I can't—so I can't change yesterday, because that's like yesterday. It's over. I'm too old for yesterday and too young for tomorrow, so I'm living now. And I have to make tomorrow.*

Participants seemed to be realistic in assessing their situations. When in a state of recovery, participants reported a strong sense of hope for the future and that they had the capacity to keep learning how to cope with their new realities:

Alisa: *Not being able to totally 100 percent accept having an illness, still. Same things, but to a lesser degree, like I have the same kind of issues, but to a less degree. Like I'm better now with these issues because I've matured and I've grown up from then. Not figuratively speaking grown up but actually, technically grown up, because when you mature, when you get to 18, 19, you're mature, you see, you do view life differently than you were 11, 10. Right? Because you're maturing, you mature.*

Conditions for Recovery: Community-Based Youth-Centred Support

Most female participants and some of the males emphasized that a key factor in their recovery and stability was that they became part of a community-based program focused on youth with mental health problems. An important aspect of this program was the "drop-in," where they could gain social support and feel they had a safe place to relate to one another:

Interviewer: *Let's pretend I attended a community-based mental health program and it's my first time, and I'm scared and I don't know what to do and I ask your advice.*
Zita: *I will say that you're safe in here. It's very safe. Whatever the problem you have, you can ask the staff, you can talk. Nobody has to know that you are talking to a staff [sic], and they will keep a secret and they will help you. In another way. And the people here are very friendly. And I, by myself, I do feel a lot of progressing ... when I came here.*

The next quote shows how the youth supported one another and built a bit of a network with one another:

Scott: *Yeah. And I was very worried about him, you know. Yeah. And I brought him home. He was rude to me but I understand him, and—*

another time, just before that, he was drinking a mickey and I dumped it out, I broke the bottle, and I just tapped it and I poured it out so he doesn't drink any more. I was worried about him. And I made him a $20 bet, if he doesn't drink 'til the end of this month, right now, I'll give him $20 and I'll keep my word, and he hasn't drinked [sic] yet.

Another youth discussed the importance of peer groups:

Alisa: *Yes, here [at the community centre for youth with mental health problems] ... just talking to—just talking to the kids, you know, talking to other people my age, a little older, a little younger than me, having— you know, relating to each other, having common ground, 'cause we both have illnesses.*

Jack underscores the importance of peer support and social acceptance and suggests that coping with mental illness in some ways has more to do with addressing and enduring the stigma, discrimination, and prejudice that accompany it.

Reintegration

The challenge of functioning in the social world becomes evident when youth need to socialize beyond the youth and mental health community centre. Participants still reported difficulty in the social world, not because of the symptoms of mental illness, but because of the label and stigma attached to mental illness. This new identity included being someone with mental health problems.

While they needed the label to access support, socially they had difficulty getting beyond the label to truly re-enter the world without being stigmatized or marginalized:

Interviewer: *But I hear what you're saying though. You're saying, if I understand you correctly, that you would like start over, without stigma ... And have a fresh start.*

Amin: *Mm-hm. But that's not now going to change, because the label is going to be there, this never change. But the stigma, sometime we can change, sometime they can't.*

Seta: *It's true, they have a saying that—to have health, good health, is actually better than to have a lot of money. In a way. Yeah.*

Reintegration: Volunteering

Young people expressed an interest in volunteering so that they could feel good about themselves by giving something back to their communities and as part of the process of reintegration. Participants who had volunteered in the past or who were currently volunteering in their communities spoke of their voluntary work as a positive experience. It gave them a chance to see and relate to others in need, and feel as though their interventions were important and appreciated. An extra advantage was that, when volunteering, the focus was not on their mental illness, but on their role as a volunteer. If this kind of opportunity were readily available and encouraged by workers and parents, it might help them in their recovery and reintegration. Two examples of how young people felt good about themselves by giving something back to the community are provided below:

Amin: *That's more kind of helpful for me, to be able to help other teenagers. But the thing is, I want to tell more teenagers not to go into the problems or, you know, like the stupid way I did ... After I got my mental illness, I want to help people, but before that, I never did to anyone.*
Alisa: *Yes, I volunteered at [name of facility]. It's a senior home, senior residence for the elderly ... they're in wheelchairs most of them, obviously. And I wheelchair them around. I did Meals on Wheels. Yeah, I gave lunch to, oh, many people, many people in the vacancies, in the apartments that they live in. And I was also—at the beginning I was doing laundry, like laundry downstairs. They needed someone to fold ... not clothes, fold towels, and all those things for the residents, and so I gave my time to the laundry, and then they put me on the 5th floor in the serious—the ward where the residents are most troubled. Like they have*

Alzheimer's. And I was with them, and that was a really good experience, because I found, like I was so giving. I wanted to help them. And I felt that I was giving them the help they wanted, like keeping them company, wheelchairing them around. Just—just keeping them company, and they'd smile at you—when you said something to them, 'cause nobody pays attention to them. The family, relatives don't really come. But there are relatives that come but not very often, and they feel, you know, one of them cries because, like she doesn't know why she cries but she cries, it's just Alzheimer's. A lot of things—different people do different—you know, act differently? So—but it was, it was a really good experience for the—I was only up on the 5th floor for a couple of weeks, but it was enough to see the whole picture of how these people need to be cared for, and loved, especially loved.

When youth are in a state of recovery, they are working on reintegrating themselves into the social world. The participants described the need to connect with other youth with mental health problems to create a sense of belonging and community. They also articulated some strategies for maintaining a sense of homeostasis, including:

- getting the right medications prescribed and taking them regularly
- finding a doctor who understands their situation
- having family support
- living at home with parents or in a comfortable independent living situation
- having community-based supports

Further, youth described the importance of having a sense of hope for the future and maintaining a positive attitude, which helps with accepting their situation.

Summary

■ THROUGH THE PROCESS of using a constant comparison methodology, four main themes emerged from the data: emergence, loss, adaptation, and recovery. Emergence represents the process of becoming mentally ill, including being labelled, stigmatized, and marginalized. The second category, loss, describes how the youth lost their sense of self or social identity as a result of the diagnosis. Adaptation involves the process the youth go through and the coping skills they develop to accept that they have a mental illness. Finally, in the recovery stage, youth re-establish a sense of self and social identity. The quotes provided by the participants support the development of these four categories.

FIVE

Understanding: Integrating the Results

Alisa: And I feel that people need to get more educated on the kind, on the kind of mental illnesses there are, in order for them not to be so scared of them. In order for them not to be afraid of the topic. Like some people, the topic, when you get on that, it's like, you know someone that's like that, it's like, yeah, I have something, I felt like telling them. Like, so what?

I N THIS CHAPTER I integrate the key findings and explore their implications. How do we understand the stages of emergence, loss, adaptation, and recovery? What are the potential effects of stigma on the recovery process for youth with mental illness? How does the interruption of developmental and identity tasks affect the recovery process? How do we understand this theoretically and as practitioners—and what do we do about it?

Integrating the Results and the Stages of Emergence, Loss, Adaptation, and Recovery

■ THE MAJOR FINDINGS in this study centre on how youth described their lived experience of mental illness and how they derived meaning in their lives given the onset of their illness, with particular emphasis on the psychosocial effects of mental illness on identity and life cycle development. The developing theory presented in this chapter represents the participants' collectively described experiences. This research was framed in the literature, which suggests that identity development and developmental or life cycle tasks are delayed or disrupted based on the onset, and ongoing experiences of, mental illness. The results of this particular sample indicate something slightly different. The data reveal that while the participants' developmental tasks and identity development were delayed and disrupted, at least by society's typical measures, these participants did meet their developmental and identity challenges. However, they did this differently through the stages of emergence, loss, adaptation, and recovery.

The details of how participants' developmental stages and adult identity formation were affected by mental illness and how milestones were achieved or delayed are woven throughout this chapter. In an approach to developing theory, the relevant literature provides a general context for what youth reported. This section presents a developing theory and a framework for understanding participants' experiences; it also explores the implications of experiencing the stages of emergence, loss, adaptation, and recovery. Further, this section discusses the implications of the key issues identified by participants regarding the achievement of their age-related developmental tasks and young adult identities in the context of having a mental health problem. A modified gender analysis attempts to explain why the results of the gender-based analysis were in some ways opposite to what might be intuitively expected for youth.

General Context

■ WHAT THE YOUTH PARTICIPANTS SAID revealed some unexpected results, such as the 100% compliance rate for taking medication along with the participants' clear concern that other youth experiencing an emerging mental illness get the right medication, at least for stabilizing purposes. This seems contrary to what many adult consumer/survivors say about medication compliance. Many say they resist this avenue because of the potential side effects, or they do not like how they feel when taking medication (M. Chappell, personal communication, January 2003).

Young adults with mental illness suggest that they need to participate actively in the larger community, feel appreciated, and be rewarded just like anyone else in society. In fact, they may have *more* need to contribute to their social environment because of their mental illness (perhaps, as one or two participants reported, because they need to prove themselves). Finishing their education, beginning a career, working, getting their own apartment, becoming independent, and volunteering are common tasks and aspirations for all youth, including, and perhaps even especially, young people with a mental illness.

Overall, the themes of stigma, labelling, and multiple losses were evident throughout the data in all four categories: emergence, loss, adaptation, and recovery. The data from youth on the theme of stigma focused on their feeling ostracized by their friends and family members, and marginalized from them and from their external psychosocial environments.

The data on the theme of labelling focused on the effects of an individual not having the capability to meet an acceptably "sick" role status as conceptualized by Talcott Parsons. Parsons indicates, for example, that the stigma associated with the onset of a mental illness implies that the illness itself is not socially acceptable; therefore, it is automatically stigmatized (Illich, 1976). The potential chronicity of mental illness does not allow individuals to recover quickly and resume their previous level of social functioning, and the ability to comply with prescribed treatment may not be consistent. All of these factors have the potential to cause loss of social support. We can see this in the theme of multiple losses, which include loss of a "normal" identity, credibility, friends, family, independence, social standing, and income ability.

Stigma is inherently complex, but it is important to understand its dynamics for youth with mental illness diagnoses so that both the social environment and the individual can move beyond the label and stigma of mental illness. Listening to youths' experiences of mental illness and understanding them within the framework presented is an important advance for informing policy work in this area. Participants were clear regarding what did or did not help them in their process of recovery.

....

Developing Theory about Youth and Mental Illness: A Framework for Understanding

■ AS EXPRESSED EARLIER IN THE BOOK, there is little data reflecting the voices of youth experiencing a mental illness. Further, there appears to be a system gap between the child and adolescent, and adult mental health service systems, which fails to address youth aged 16 to 24 and their specific mental health needs. If this gap were addressed, professionals could assist youth in recovering from their mental illnesses and, at the same time, through early and accurate interventions, help them address the delay in developmental tasks.

By exploring some of the identity-related and psychosocial needs of youth with mental illness, this research adds knowledge that will help professionals help youth in their recovery processes. It is clear that we can derive important program and policy implications from learning more about the self-perceptions and experiences of youth with mental illness.

Connecting Themes and Categories

The connection between the themes and the categories shows that acquiring a mental illness creates a problematic social image. The individual experiences social stigma because of a label and is subsequently marginalized by the social world. The illness then defines and distinguishes the individual in relation to his social identity. The label of mental illness becomes the defining point of the self in relation to the social world, including a person's external identity and image and internal emotional responses to the social realities of stigma, labelling, and subsequent social and functional losses. This leaves youth with a sense of existential struggle to find new meaning in life from a place of disadvantage.

The themes of stigma, labelling, and loss represent how youth interpret themselves in relation to the world and their reactions to it. Mental illness becomes the means through which these youth communicate and understand their worlds. These themes are evident in all four categories analyzed from the data and therefore form the substructure of the developing theory that follows.

A Developing Theory

The meaning of mental illness to youth, the concept of the "interrupted self," or the "mentally ill self," as evidenced by the data in this study, can be stated as follows:

Illness considered as process helps us understand the experience of youth being diagnosed with a mental illness. We can view this process through a set of stages—emergence, loss, adaptation, and recovery—that youth move through in a dynamic manner at different times during their illness. Understanding the onset of mental illness in young people as a process is an important means by which to consider how youth adapt and change in relation to their internal and external circumstances of biological and social changes.

Overall, youth with mental illness experience their social world as a place where they are labelled and stigmatized. Youth with mental illness are required to negotiate the world through mental illness, which is present in all aspects of their internal physiological and external social experiences. The social and biological reality of mental illness creates the meaning of their worlds; that meaning then defines their internal and external environments. Therefore, what they experience externally has the potential to be expressed internally through a developmental disruption. Youth experience the effects of the social construction of mental illness and subsequently may experience the reality of an "interrupted-self." When mental illness leads to an interrupted-self, there are negative identity and developmental implications for social maturation and development. This social reality is further complicated by youth having no control over the biological facts of acquiring the illness. Therefore, initially youth are victim to their illness both biologically and socially and must learn how to cope with this reality state, or way of being, and recover.

....

Considerations for Practice

■ A NUMBER OF ASSUMPTIONS are threaded throughout the theory stated above, including the following:

- The stages emergence, loss, adaptation, and recovery are not static, nor can they be applied linearly. The stages are dynamic and can move forward or backward or in multiple directions at any point in time.

- An individual may progress and regress, as each person has a unique set of experiences, strengths, and weaknesses, which impact how the person moves through the processes.

- Because of the nature of mental illness, clinical and/or social stability is not a static state, and stability cannot be guaranteed and fixed by intervention alone. Thus, we need to understand the illness process as a dynamic state that requires the individual to respond. This dynamic state will challenge the social environment in which the individual is situated and interacts. It then becomes necessary for the social environment to acknowledge and react. In other words, the individual will affect the social group around him and the group will influence the individual.

The Stages of Emergence, Loss, Adaptation, and Recovery

■ THE STAGES of emergence, loss, adaptation, and recovery emerged from the data. In the next section, I discuss these stages in the context of youth with mental illness and their capacity to meet age-related developmental tasks and young adult identity formation. The categories and analysis apply to the participants in this study, but further research is needed to reveal whether these are generalizable to other youth with mental illness.

Emergence

This study revealed several aspects of the emergence and process of becoming mentally ill in the context of adolescence, transition, and young adulthood. Youth are quite aware of the discrepancy between what they know as their reality and the social reality they are forced to negotiate within this new altered identity, an identity that now includes a mental illness. No longer can they meld in with the rest of their peers or family members. On some level, these youth know they have a different status in the social hierarchy. In some cases, they are desperately trying to negotiate their social realities, clinging to their much-needed former senses of self, yet at the same time witnessing that without much control, these former selves become completely "emerged" in the social and physiological process of illness. They have become full citizens of this other place, the kingdom of the ill (Sontag, 1989).

The process of an individual losing her sense of social identity is a devastating plummet from which some do not recover (McGorry et al., 1996). Because society is interactive in nature, the loss of self through the stigma of mental illness is particularly difficult. A destruction occurs in the receiver of stigma (Goffman, 1963), and a new "frame" emerges by which the individual is now viewed, judged, and categorized. Participants reported that their families became overprotective and inadvertently undermined their ability to acquire and develop life skills. On the other hand, some individuals experienced being marginalized, isolated, and ostracized by both families and friends and therefore did not benefit from any sort of protection from either group.

In terms of life cycle tasks and identity formation, it is clear that the participants experienced difficult biological and emotional effects because of the onset of mental illness. Participants experienced having an altered identity, which, though difficult, still constituted a process of evolution. Being challenged with a mental illness, participants were forced to deal with personal tragedy but survived the process. Their developmental process was delayed due to the interruption of the illness. The emergence process, while inherently negative, changed the participants' worlds at this stage. However, the positive aspect of the stage of emergence is that participants were able to identify that there was something wrong that needed to be addressed. We can view this acknowledgement of needing help as the beginning of independence, or self-responsibility, which fits within the developmental stage of becoming a young adult. Comparatively, typical age group peers are expected to have the skills to identify whether they require medical assistance and seek help. Therefore, in this example the inference is that both groups meet developmental milestones, just differently.

Loss

When examining the literature and listening to participants' interviews, it appears that individuals experiencing mental illness lose their prior identity as "normal" and become "citizens of illness" (Sontag, 1989). This loss of identity is partly caused by the mental illness (i.e., the symptoms), and in a more devastating way is caused by being marginalized and stigmatized by the larger societal group. Stigmatization of persons with a mental illness is done to individuals who are essentially innocent of any wrongdoing. These individuals have no control over what is experienced. They are people who have an illness and are in need of help. However, because the illness is mental, they become victim to society's judgment. As a result, they sustain a social loss over which they have no control. It remains a challenge as to how youth can remedy their loss. The loss of multiple aspects of identity is of particular significance in this age population because it involves both the stage of identity formation and achievement, and the transition to young adulthood. To negotiate and achieve the status of young adult, a person must first have a solid sense of himself, which is usually achieved by possessing an internal locus of control (Marcia, 1966).

Research purports that the harder a person works to resolve her identity crisis, the stronger a sense of self the person will have (Marcia, 1966). That said, the participants reported working *very* hard at resolving their problems in living. Overall, they were motivated as a group to succeed at life cycle tasks. Achieving these developmental identity tasks is difficult for a typical youth without mental illness. When a person experiencing a mental illness, who is also going through the typical transition of adolescence to young adulthood, has to deal with a major disruption because of the illness, that person's natural progression or evolution is disrupted. Participants demonstrated a lost opportunity for typical identity formation as evidenced by disruption at school, loss of friends, and disrupted academic function, which further disrupted and delayed their maturation rate as a group. However, as stated earlier, they were motivated to work hard to overcome these problems. According to Marcia (1966), this group may have a good chance of overcoming the age-stage related issues, notwithstanding mental illness, because of their motivation to work hard, pursue wellness, and achieve personal goals.

Based on these measures, we can say that these youth have indeed achieved the developmental tasks involved in creating a young adult identity. The participants experienced and survived biological and psychosocial challenges that most of their peers may never have to face. While participants in this study may remain interrupted in forming intimate relationships, they have been able to pursue career and educational goals within an adult framework. Even in the context of extreme loss and disruption, the participants realized the importance of securing their futures. So it is important for practitioners working with youth to understand health as a dynamic state that has the potential to be restored. This understanding could begin to shift our attention away from what is lost, such as a typical life stage process of identity formation, to what could potentially be gained, restored, or compensated for (Neuman, 1982). Perhaps we can then view this loss as an experience that places individuals in a position to adapt or change. As a result, individuals are forced to change based on the intense circumstances, which may cause them to mature at a more rapid pace than their healthier peers.

Adaptation

Instead of using negative vocabulary when referring to mental illness, it might be more productive if professionals considered using the term mental wellness. They could then assess the individual on a continuum of wellness: "Attitudes can help you to be well or can lead you to being ill" (Moller & Murphy, 1998, pp. 1-8). From Neuman's perspective, the health care system aims to help individuals and families "maintain a maximum level of total wellness by purposeful interventions" through a "reduction of stress factors and adverse conditions which either affect or could affect optimal functioning" (1982, p. 12). In addition, Neuman (1982) views the individual in the light of four variables: physiological, psychological, socio-cultural, and developmental. These variables and the physical environment affect the individual's ability to adapt. Therefore, when assessing a young person's needs and planning for individualized treatment and paths to recovery, professionals need to consider a holistic approach that includes the physical *and* social environments. The level of functioning and the attitudes of the individual and those around him are key variables in the rehabilitation process. Framing a wellness continuum of health and promoting a positive attitude for the individual and those around him will help the young person adapt to his new state, which includes mental illness.

In this study, adaptation became the process by which youth were challenged to adjust to a new state of being, as few other options existed. They were challenged to overcome their previous social reality and former selves and adapt or metamorphose into a self-identified person with an illness or problem. The mental health problem mediated or infiltrated all aspects of the social and biological lives of those interviewed. The data reveal that the resilient or resourceful young person will seek help, or an aware family will help the youth access mental health services, to reach a state of stabilization or homeostasis. This adaptive or new state will not be like the previous functional state. Rather, this adaptive state will be a changed or altered state that includes a redefined self-identity, state of wellness, and level of social and biological functioning and self-understanding.

These data show individuals experiencing themselves on a continuum of adaptive states. For example, some female participants felt that their social worlds were more difficult since being diagnosed. On the other hand, many females felt their self-image had improved. Females in this group found it hard to adapt socially but discovered that they were able to adapt their self-image (in a positive way) since feeling stable, and had a sense of relief in knowing what was wrong with them. Because they were knowledgeable about having an illness, it gave them a renewed sense of control, as they were able to seek intervention. Therefore, we could conclude that their social functioning would improve the longer they maintained a stable state, given that stability allowed an improved self-image. This stability and improved self-image allowed the participants to deal with the developmental task of moving to a state of self-acceptance and taking on the adult role of accepting their health state, seeking out the resources to deal with their problems, and relying on their own initiative to adapt.

Recovery

Olivia: *I own the illness; the illness does not own me.*

In the quote above, Olivia is stating that it is really not a cure that makes the difference; rather, a state of mind is what matters—taking control over a situation in which she once felt almost a victim. Now she has control and the illness is just something she must deal with. This is critical in the recovery process, as recovery is a lifelong state of balancing dimensions of wellness to maintain a state of homeostasis or satisfactory functionality.

People with mental illness comment on the importance of peer groups in their recovery process as a place to be understood without feeling judged negatively. This environment then helps them help others by giving them the confidence to share what coping strategies have worked in gaining control of their illness (Leavey, 2003, 2005; Moller & Murphy, 1997; Rice & Moller, 2006; Wahl, 1999). Recovery is a state whereby the young person with a mental illness has productively passed through a series of experiences in relation to the social stigma and physiological reality of the illness. The young people interviewed described losing their pre-illness sense of self, becoming labelled as deviant or different, acquiring a spoiled identity, becoming more dependent on their family, losing friends, and feeling that they had become outsiders to their former worlds.

However, in managing the process of the adaptation to a new state of being or an alternative state of wellness, these individuals also described the potential to re-emerge with a new identity, or an identity that integrated their mental states. As revealed in the data, the young people interviewed learned to cope with their experiences of internal and external stigma as well as changes in their biological states and functioning, and moved on to a new level of living. This is supported by Neuman's belief that stressors are both beneficial and noxious (1996). Depending on a person's skills and support systems (i.e., family, friends, and mental health services), the person can adapt to circumstances and can create a stable sense of wellness (Moller & Murphy, 1998).

Recovery is a process by which the young person is challenged to make his way back to health. Stigma has now become a filter or funnel through which the young person now sees his reality. Because of the effects of stigma, getting to and/or maintaining the recovery phase makes dealing with a mental illness even more complicated. Therefore, it becomes paramount that the proper supports and services, family and peer education, peer support, and ways to find a meaningful existence (e.g., through work and love) (Smelser & Erickson, 1980) are available and accessible to youth with mental illness.

Part of the process of recovery is interactive. It must involve a team of people who support and understand youth with mental health problems and the challenges they are facing. For youth experiencing mental illness, there are many meanings associated with being chronically ill. These meanings need to be updated and rooted in the realities that young people face. Their development and achievement of the milestones of young adulthood depend on the opportunities available to them, just as for any other youth in society. Work, love, family, friends, career, education, and sexual intimacy are all typical experiences available to most youth. Most youth in this study, both male and female, reported getting their social meaning from these kinds of experiences. When deprived, they plummeted further into a state of despair.

That said, the ways in which individuals with mental illness cope with stigma is a key factor in whether they recover. In a nation-wide study conducted by Wahl and associates (1999), the researchers asked 100 individuals how they addressed the issue of stigma and how they coped with it. Many participants stated that they used the coping strategy of concealment: they were cautious about who they told and did not reveal their mental health histories on job applications or licence forms, or to any other agencies that might have the power to use the information to stigmatize them (Wahl, 1999). This coping strategy is one of the ways that people with mental illness deal with the stigma.

Maintaining Conditions for Recovery

In terms of psychosocial needs, participants were clear about their needs and what could help other youth experiencing mental health problems. They stated that they need early intervention to be diagnosed with a label or title, for this will allow them and their families to access expert, timely, and appropriate treatment (especially medication). It is well documented that the earlier the intervention, the better the long-term prognosis (Macnaughton, 1997; Malla, 1999; McGorry, 1992; McGorry et al., 1996). They also need a stress-free, non-stigmatized environment with a youth-centred program where youth have peers and a general sense of safety and acceptance. Public health education is needed to help society understand mental illness in such a way that it becomes assimilated and normalized. As a result, the onset of mental illness would be treated like any other health issue, and in the normal course of events, an individual would feel free to concentrate on the mental problem and openly seek help and receive support. The individual would no longer be required to accept devastating social losses by hiding the facts to avoid being stigmatized.

....

Integration and Implications of Key Findings

The Developmental Stages

As stated earlier, working through developmental milestones is the challenge of all youth. These transitions tend to be difficult, even for the most typical or stable youth. For youth experiencing mental health problems, these typical developmental milestones are often delayed or disrupted (McGorry et al.,

1996). Because these developmental issues can also affect basic mental health functioning, we can reasonably assume that the developmental tasks of social connection, work, educational achievement, independence from family, and establishing an intimate relationship will be disrupted for young people with mental illness. However, we have learned that at least for this sample, the youth were aware of what they were going through and felt capable of articulating their needs. Perhaps further study is needed at this particular stage to measure how individuals make decisions regarding their mental health care needs and whether those decisions are health and age appropriate.

Further, this research showed that youth with mental illness in some senses do meet their milestones, at least eventually. It seems that, as the literature states, the timing of meeting typical milestones, including getting work, graduating from high school, entering college or university, and forming intimate relationships, was delayed. However, these participants were ahead of their healthier peers in terms of having to deal with a mental illness, and therefore life-related issues were far more complex. The participants learned how to negotiate institutions and systems, make treatment decisions about medication and hospital admissions, articulate their needs, cope with adversity, loss, and grieving, and, finally, recover. It appears that, compared with their typical peers, the participants were more advanced developmentally in these areas, and that through the stages and processes of becoming mentally ill, they had in fact formed an adult identity. Therefore, a youth-centred mental health care system is very important to help youth meet their developmental and identity needs, as well as their medical needs. The need for youth peer programs becomes obvious when helping youth with mental illness meet their need to form social relationships and to have a place to develop and work on their life cycle goals.

Potential Developmental Effect of Stigma on Youth with Mental Illness

The literature indicates that it is important to see stigma from a number of different perspectives, such as spoiled character, media, and negative mental illness jargon. It also shows how insidious stigma is in our culture and how negative it is with respect to the individual experiencing mental illness (Wahl, 1999). Further, understanding the social aspects and effects of mental illness is important because ultimately these effects have potential developmental implications for youth experiencing mental illness. The social experience of mental illness is significant because of the potential negative effects that stigma may have on the prognosis of the biological aspects of the mental illness process (McGorry et al., 1996). Potentially, stress could accelerate or worsen the biological aspect of the mental illness, which in turn could disrupt the developmental process by taking the youth's focus away from typical task achievement and instead placing it on surviving the illness. Social stigma disrupts, spoils, or alters the course of a person's life and damages some of the healthier options of career, family, and education available to others. The disruption and multiple loss of being stigmatized can be conceptualized as the symptomatology of the social disease, which accompanies mental illness.

The biggest challenge for participants seems to be dealing with the stigma attached to having a mental illness. Stigma is the major barrier to participants' ability to reintegrate into the social world, based on social reactions to their mental illnesses. It leaves them feeling "different," the antithesis of what youth want to feel at this developmental stage. Youth need to be integrated and attached socially so that they may move into adulthood feeling a sense of autonomy, attachment, and productivity. These are the building blocks to developmental and identity achievement of young adulthood (Erikson, 1980). When these developmental building blocks are interrupted, youth may be left vulnerable to struggling with a sense of marginalization and isolation from family, friends, and society. These issues pose difficult and complex policy issues in developing mental health supports and services that address stigma and the related issues.

Money Matters

A few participants mentioned financial support as an issue. This was likely because they were living on government benefits either independently or in a group home situation. As a result, they had some experience with trying to survive on their own as young adults. Other participants were still living at home or had other means of financial support in addition to disability benefits. However, these data show that all participants were hoping to establish a career path, acknowledging the need to make an independent living at some point.

Transition-aged young people with a mental illness may be so preoccupied with surviving their illnesses that they are unaware of their longer-term socio-economic needs. Remaining stable in the illness is perhaps their first priority, but the data show that all of the youth interviewed had ideas, dreams, and desires for careers and wanted to finish their education to achieve those career goals. Class status and the ability to make a living are important, given that these are two pillars of the social determinants of health (Health Canada, 1999a). Because youth with a mental illness are dealing with a chronic health problem, they need to concentrate on such things as proper nutrition, sufficient sleep, regular exercise, and appropriate medication. If transition-aged youth do not have adequate financial resources, their concentration turns to survival, not health, which makes it that much harder for them to attain their developmental milestones of independence, intimacy, and comfort in adult roles.

The high incidence of psychiatric disorders in homeless youth, as well as high rates of childhood problems and mental health problems (Craig & Hodson, 1998), further suggest a critical relationship between access to housing and the ability to maintain it for transition-aged youth. "More and more, our nation is becoming class-segregated. The poor live with and among the poor ... without adequate shelter, food, or health care" (hooks, 2000b, p. 2). Any visible difference, such as mental illness, makes it easy to identify and exclude the stigmatized individual and in effect segregates that person from sharing in wealth or being of any class other than disadvantaged, impoverished, and dispossessed (hooks, 2000a, 2000b).

Pat Capponi, a mental illness consumer/survivor, psychiatric advocate, and writer, has described her long-standing relationship with the psychiatric world. A consequence of this relationship, in part, is living below or close to the poverty line. In her book *Dispatches from the Poverty Line* (1997), she describes being a psychiatric survivor living in a state of subsistence and the challenges it creates. She specifically elaborates on the concept of poverty, upon which many psychiatric survivors spend immense energy. It is an issue that many of these youth will face if they are not integrated into the larger societal context by developing financial independence. If financial independence is not an option, Capponi, a professional survivor, describes a bleak existence:

> Planning in the face of expected disaster. I immediately determine to put myself on a rationing regime ... It's not like I haven't been down-and-out poor before. Not like I'm a stranger to hunger. The first thing I have to do is get my stomach used to less. The worst thing about hunger is the headaches it gives you, which for me always threaten to escalate into migraines, and I can't afford $100 for six pills, the cost of the miracle medication. Drinking lots of water can fool the stomach into believing it's had more than it really has [sic] had. Step one. Step two. Ration cigarettes. Put an open pack in the fridge instead of right where I can see and reach for them without thinking. Step three. Go out immediately and convert the bulk of my remaining cash into money orders made out to my landlord: don't trust that common sense will prevail over immediate need. I've had to make the choice a number of times in my life, whether to eat or keep a roof over my head. (1997, p. 7)

Providing appropriate job training and education to meet the need of financial independence becomes an important issue for health planners and policy-makers to include in their systems designs in meeting the overall mental health needs of young people. This would help ensure they have every opportunity for the best possible chance of gaining a sense of recovery, maintaining it, and achieving a sense of social reintegration. Being able to achieve an income and a work role could reduce or even mitigate the chances of developing a long-standing relationship with poverty and a marginalized social status. Reducing the socio-economic challenges also reduces stressors related to poverty, thereby improving opportunities for better mental health (Health Canada, 1999a).

Understanding Gender

Although gender was not the major focus of this research, some gender differences and similarities were identified that are worth comment. First, females tended to have different diagnoses than males. For example, females had more internally located mental illnesses such as anxiety, depression, and post-traumatic stress disorder, whereas males had diagnoses such as conduct disorder, psychosis, schizophrenia, and bipolar experiences. As Offord and colleagues (1987) indicated, diagnostic criteria seem to be applied differently to males versus females. Is this a true clinical picture, or is it how we as humans are socialized to interpret male and female behaviour?

In this research, males and females placed different amounts of importance on social role versus family role. Female participants were more concerned about their social identities with work and friends; males were more interested in their family role function. In addition, females were more likely to be independent of their families, whereas males were more likely to want the approval of their families and were more emotionally dependent on them for direction and compliance with treatment. At first glance, this finding seems counterintuitive. It seems that male participants (at least at this stage) were much more financially dependent on their families than were female participants. Further, families seemed more willing to support male participants than their female counterparts. It may be that males are less developmentally mature and less able to take on an adult personification. Further study in this area would be helpful in terms of tailoring programming to deal with the psychosocial differences by understanding the developmental levels of males and females.

Most female participants were diagnosed around the age of 14, and the diagnoses seemed to be more consistent and stable; males were diagnosed younger and seemed to have much more variation in their diagnostic labels over time. Are females more accepting of a diagnostic label because of a greater need to be socially accepted and compliant? Are physicians less willing to apply a diagnostic label to males, perhaps viewing their behaviour as more of a stage that the male youth is going through? An interesting speculation regarding the average age of onset of mental illness for females (14 years) and the ensuing depression and anxiety is that there may be a hormonal link between puberty and the onset of depression and/or anxiety. It may be that a similar link exists for pubescent boys, since they exhibit more "acting out" types of behaviours (Offord et al., 1987).

The most common similarities between males and females were compliance with medication, the belief that individuals need an accurate diagnostic label, and the need to finish their education. Some gender differences need further research to grasp the relevant implications for treatment and programming and the long-term effects of these differences—for example, on income ability, independent living, self-responsibility, and biological and long-term treatment prognoses. The overall categories, themes, and subthemes were identified by both males and females with regard to their experiences; however, how they applied to each gender differed in some circumstances.

....

Summary

■ THE THEMES of stigma, labelling, and multiple losses were evident throughout the data in all four categories: emergence, loss, adaptation, and recovery. These categories form the substructure of the proposed developing theory. In addition, the categories help us understand the illness process by providing a framework and context from which to interpret what is happening to individuals experiencing mental illness and how to facilitate their recovery.

SIX

Where Are We and Where Do We Go from Here?

Carrie: *Just don't look at anything bad, just keep on going, keep your high hopes and just keep on going and just don't look around people around you ... or don't look at them or their habits, because—just do what you think you have to do and don't get caught up. [pause] Don't think of anything negative too much.*

THIS FINAL CHAPTER provides a brief overview of the current gaps in service delivery, discusses the significance of treatment interventions, and in particular speaks about the fundamentals of and need for early identification and intervention. The chapter concludes with a section on considerations and implications for future program and policy design.

....

Gap in Service Delivery

■ CANADIAN MENTAL HEALTH SYSTEMS have historically had a deficit of youth-focused mental health services. This is evidenced by gaps in medical services and social programs available to young adults (National Early Psychosis Program, 1997). Further, there have been few or no transitional services available between the child and adult mental health care systems for youth going from one system to another (District Health Councils of Southwestern Ontario, 1996; Leavey et al., 2000; Thames Valley District Health Council, 1997; Vancouver/Richmond Health Board, 1998). Service providers who work with transition-aged youth with mental illness clearly identify the lack of service integration and coordination for this population, addressing specific risk factors as outlined earlier (Central Toronto Youth Services, 2002).

Internationally, there appears to be a dearth of health care services and community supports available for transition-aged youth, of the sort that would that provide early intervention aimed at alleviating potential developmental delays and interrupted young adult identity achievement (Early Psychosis Prevention and Intervention Centre, 2000; Malla, Norman, & Voruganti, 1999; McGorry, 1992). Finally, educators believe that though there are a number of school-based initiatives, current approaches "are not dealing with the problems systematically and effectively" (Santor, Short, & Ferguson, 2009, p. 8).

Making visible the resilience and struggle of young people as they move through the system is of direct relevance to Canadian research and practice. Though there has been a lack of youth-centred mental health services in the past, this appears to be changing. There are currently a number of major Canadian initiatives in progress to address the mental health of young people. Selected initiatives are briefly described below:

- *The Jack Project.* This charitable organization was founded in 2010 in memory of Jack Windeler, a student at Queen's University who tragically died by suicide. The organization focuses on province-wide workshops, investments in youth-oriented technology, and a national student-led mental health summit. (www.thejackproject.org)

- *Mental Health Commission of Canada (MHCC).* This organization offers direction on how to address child and youth mental health issues. It initiated a project to better understand the service delivery gaps that exist for youth experiencing mental health problems. The organization also engages directly with young people to develop programs and strategies. The MHCC has implemented a national anti-stigma initiative, identifying youth as an important target group for research. (www.mentalhealthcommission.ca)

- *Transformational Research in Adolescent Mental Health* (TRAM). A joint partnership between the Canadian Institutes of Health Research and the Graham Boeckh Foundation, TRAM focuses on bringing fundamental change to Canadian youth mental health care. TRAM is working with patients and families, policy-makers, researchers, service providers, and community organizations to implement evidence-based findings. (tramcan.ca/home)

- *Children's Health Policy Centre.* This interdisciplinary research group aims to improve children's and youth's social and emotional health and reduce health disparities starting in childhood. The group works to create connections between research and policy, promote effective programs and services, and monitor progress toward improving the lives of children. (childhealthpolicy.ca)

- *Mind Your Mind.* This not-for-profit mental health program works with youth and professionals to develop reliable and relevant resources. The program uses current evidence and research to reduce the stigma associated with mental illness and increase access to and use of community support. (www.mindyourmind.ca)

- *Teen Mental Health.* The goal of this organization is to improve the mental health of youth using scientific evidence and knowledge. The organization uses the best evidence available to develop programs, publications, tools, and resources to enhance understanding of adolescent mental health and mental disorders. (teenmentalhealth.org)

- *Evergreen.* This national-level health framework was designed using online technologies to be a resource for provincial and territorial governments and institutions. Its goal is to help policy-makers, planers, and health care providers to create, implement, and review mental health policies, plans, programs, and services (Kutcher & McLuckie, 2011). (http://www.forcesociety.com/sites/default/files/Evergreen_Framework_English_July_2010_final.pdf)

....

Significance of Early Intervention

■ EARLY INTERVENTION for young people experiencing an emerging mental illness is critical in the recovery and stabilization process as well as in fostering a positive prognostic outcome (Macnaughton, 1997, 1999; Malla et al., 1999; McGorry, 1992; McGorry et al., 1996). In particular, delayed treatment intervention is a strong predictor of poor outcomes for individuals with emerging schizophrenia. A delay in diagnosis and treatment can lead to interruptions in education and work as well as a slower and less complete recovery (Lincoln & McGorry, 1995). Early intervention partnered with home-based care (where abuse is not present in the home), supported by community physician treatment intervention, is a strong indicator of a more complete and long-term recovery (McGorry et al., 1996). Programs that include stress or anger management, reduce violence and substance abuse, and promote prosocial behaviour "both facilitate the development of good mental health and prevent the development of disorders and difficulties" (Santor, Short, & Ferguson, 2009, p. 8).

....

Implications and Suggestions for Testing the Theoretical Framework

Clinical/Environmental Considerations

To understand the mental health needs of young people with mental health problems in the context of experiencing stigma, prejudice, and discrimination, it is important to remember that adolescence and young adulthood are characterized by periods of transition and reorganization. Assessing the mental health of adolescents and young adults in the context of the social determinants of health—which include the familial, social, and cultural expectations for age-appropriate thoughts, emotions, and behaviours (Health Canada 1999a)—is critical to their adaptation to adulthood. It is vital to understand the challenges of this age and stage to gauge the enormous difficulties faced by young people with mental illnesses in their journeys of survival and their achievement of identity, psychosocial development, and intimacy needs. This is a critical time in young people's psychosocial development as well as a critical time in the development of a mental illness. Young people facing psychosis and other mental health problems could experience a permanent disruption in their ability to function (Kessler, Forster, Saunders, & Stang, 1995) because of a serious illness that has social and biological consequences.

There is no more powerful barrier to success in society than the social stigma placed on individuals with a chronic illness that affects either social function or social identity (Davidson, 2003; Davidson & Strauss, 1992; Goffman, 1963; Leavey, 2003; Sontag, 1989). They alone must carry the burden of their loss, with no shield of protection. They are truly vulnerable in these emotional and physiological states. Given the lived experience of youth with mental illness, controlling the effects of this reality and the internal emotional states that result is often fundamental in their battle to adapt or fight back to a state of wellness (Davidson, 2003; Leavey, 2005; Murphy & Moller, 2006). However, the resulting emotional effects of stigma may never be mediated or resolved and unfortunately can become a lifetime of constant struggle (Capponi, 1997).

It is particularly important to start with the lived experience of young people themselves (Davidson, 2003; Leavey, 2003, 2005; Moller & Murphy, 1997; Rice & Moller, 2006). Recent reports such as *Out of the Shadows at Last* support the notion of typifying or normalizing mental illness through statements such as "people who are living with mental illness and addiction must be accorded respect and consideration equal to those given to people affected by physical illnesses" (Kirby & Keon, 2006, p. 5). These statements go a long way to supporting Sontag's (1989) notion that normalizing previously stigmatized illnesses so that they are accepted as "just an illness" will help demystify and destigmatize those affected by mental illnesses. It is therefore critical to reach out to typical youth in a way that is aligned with their developmental stage by understanding that they must learn how to discern group belonging and identification of difference. It is almost their "job" at this stage of development to "reject" that which seems odd or different from them. It seems that a key way to resolve the chasm between youth with mental illness and their typical peers, to reduce the fear factor, and to potentially change the stereotypes long associated with mental illness, is to reach out through the media and other methods of public awareness.

One very good example of this public education and outreach is Dr. Patrick McGorry's program ORYGEN in Australia. During the research for this book, some young people in Dr. McGorry's program reported that they felt less stigmatization now than before because of public awareness. In fact, some reported that their typical peers thought it almost "cool" to "get a psychosis." Through changes in perceptions and attitudes, modern views can change, thus improving the experience of people with mental illness in terms of quality and opportunity. There is hope that a person can recover not only from the biological illness itself but also perhaps from the experience of prejudice and the social disorder of stigma, unwittingly bestowed by peers and society.

The proposed theoretical framework of the stages (emergence, loss, adaptation, and recovery) of youth becoming mentally ill, losing their identities, adapting to the new state, and re-emerging with a new social identity, needs to be developed more thoroughly. Although testing included youth from Canada, Australia, and the United States, as well as different cultures and classes, the results are still not generalizable due to small sample size and methodology. Broader research and testing would allow an understanding of the impact of socio-economic status, cultural differences, and urban and rural differences, and their impact on psychosocial and biological experiences of mental illness. Further testing should also focus on capturing and comparing the impact these external influences have on developmental achievements and internal emotional functioning. More data testing of this theory could improve understanding of the meaning of mental illness for young people and their life-stage and developmental needs.

If this framework and theory are found to be relevant or beneficial in other places, it may reveal the importance of, for instance, the relationship between mental illness and socio-economic or cultural factors. For example, does mental illness become less visible the more money a person has? If so, what effects do socio-economic factors have on the biology of illness? Are there fewer triggers for depression when there are lower stress levels? It would be helpful to explore cross-culturally whether youth with mental health problems experience similar themes, and what the differences are.

Exploring how this theory affects youth identity and developmental stages could contribute to the body of knowledge by revealing the meaning of mental illness for youth through a common reference point. This reference point—understanding youth with mental health problems through emergency, loss, adaptation, and recovery—may be a way to understand how youth develop their adult identities and meet their age-related milestones. Future testing would also, perhaps, allow this recovery model/framework to be developed further. For example, how do the concepts of resiliency and adjustment fit into this framework or perhaps add to it? Finally, the theory discovered in this study on the "interrupted-self" stages of a mental illness framework has the potential to stimulate researchers to test its generalizability in different geographical locations, cultures, and groups.

....

Adaptation: A Conceptual Approach

■ MAINTAINING A SENSE OF EQUILIBRIUM when mental illness disrupts both the internal and external world of the individual can be a challenge, but it is not impossible. In part, equilibrium is affected by how the individual sees herself, alone and in relation to her social world. How she defines the stressor is also a factor in promoting wellness or illness. Counselling, drug treatment intervention, family support, peer support, acceptable living conditions, economic capacity, and education, as well as gender, age, and self-image, all influence an individual's adaptive state. How we frame psychosis and other mental health problems directly affects a person's psychological ability to adapt and may in fact affect the length of time it takes to reconstitute a homeostatic state (Moller & Murphy, 1998; Neuman, 1982).

For example, Neuman defines wellness as a state of inertness free of disrupting needs, and illness as a state of needs yet to be satisfied.

A conceptual approach to understanding how young people adapt to their chronic mental illness is critical to understanding the interrelationships and interplay between the person and his internal biological and emotional, and external social and physical, environments. A Darwinian view of evolutionary adaptation proposes that humans from the beginning of time have adapted to their worlds, from the perspective of both the internal and external environments (Mahoney, 1991). Whether adaptation is positive or negative depends on the biological and social determinants surrounding and within the individual (Neuman, 1982). To understand and help people adapt to difficult challenges, it is important to have a sense of individuals as a whole, of how they interact with their internal and external environments, and the strengths and challenges they might bring to the healing or adapting process.

In her Health Care Systems Model, Betty Neuman (1982) does precisely that: looks at the individual as a whole, objectively observing stressors through a neutral lens. Neuman believes that stressors are both beneficial and noxious. Depending on a person's skills, experiences, and environments, individuals experience each type of stressor differently. According to a holistic view of health, the individual should be assessed in her natural presenting state and considered as part of a larger system. In other words, "Homeostasis is a state of balance requiring energy exchanges whereby a person is able to adequately adapt to stressors and regain an optimal state of health following a reaction to a stressor and thus preserve her/his system integrity" (Neuman, 1982, p. 9).

What if we used different language when referring to mental illness? What if professionals considered mental wellness and the location of the individual they were assessing on a continuum of wellness? "Attitudes can help you to be well or can lead you to being ill" (Moller & Murphy, 1998, pp. 1–8). From Neuman's perspective, the health care system aims to help individuals and families "maintain a maximum level of total wellness by purposeful interventions" through a "reduction of stress factors and adverse conditions which either affect or could affect optimal functioning" (1982, p. 12). She views the individual through four variables: physiological, psychological, socio-cultural, and developmental. These variables and the physical environment affect the individual's ability to adapt. Therefore, when assessing a young person's needs, we need to consider a holistic approach and the physical environment. The level of functioning and the attitudes of the individual and those around him are key variables in the rehabilitation process. Framing a wellness continuum of health and promoting a positive attitude for the individual and those around him will help the young person adapt to his new state, which includes a mental illness.

Adaptive states are the ways in which people learn to accept and cope with change in their lives. Adaptation is an important part of maturation, not only for the individual but also for the community and the society in which she lives. Moving out of the family home, obtaining work, changing jobs, losing a job, the onset of a serious illness, death, and divorce are some of the things to which individuals must adjust, often radically. How a person responds and adapts to change is important to them and to the social and institutional settings in which they reside (Levinson, 1980). The elements of adaptation, such as coping, responding, and adjusting, are influenced by the event, the social context in which the event occurs, and the individual's characteristics, such as their skills, beliefs, and motives (Levinson, 1980). Internal and external determinants combine to have an impact on the individual's ability to adapt to and cope with change.

....

Recovery and Wellness

■ RECOVERY AND WELLNESS models suggest that individuals who are experiencing mental illness use their strengths and challenges to develop a plan that involves strategies for coping (Wahl, 1999). This is critical in recovery because it promotes a sense of agency, control, empowerment, and active participation in a person's care and life.

Professionals, policy-makers, and health authorities in North America are encouraging a paradigm shift that, in addition to or integrated with the biomedical view, considers the social determinants of health when assessing individuals with mental illness (National Institute of Mental Health, 1990).

For example, Health Canada has identified 12 determinants of social health, including income and social status, employment, education, social environments, physical environments, healthy child development, personal health practices and coping skills, health services, social support networks, biology and genetic endowment, gender, and culture (Health Canada, 1999a).

We can use the social determinants model to closely examine the strategies of health promotion and prevention. The practice of maintaining individuals in the community so that they remain integrated with their social support systems addresses much more of the person's whole life than traditional biomedical treatment. This approach acknowledges that all individuals are a part of a larger social and environmental system that affects their internal and external states of wellness and illness. Assessing individuals in their environmental systems helps ensure a holistic view (Moller & Murphy, 1998; Neuman, 1982; Wahl, 1999). Focusing on strengths and abilities "urges us to remember that those with psychiatric disorders are not merely passive victims of their diseases; instead, they can be (and many are) active managers, searching for and trying out strategies to lessen the impact of adverse circumstances and finding ways with their lives despite the obstacles they face" (Wahl, 1999, p. 143).

....

Implications and Suggestions for Future Program and Policy Design

■ PROFESSIONALS working with people who have mental illnesses need to know how individuals cope and what strengths they possess that promote their personal healing processes. Empowering consumers to trust and rely on their own abilities, along with whatever professional support (if any) they choose, helps the mental health consumer to function and then to relay successes to others experiencing mental illness. For example, one participant commented on his desire to help other teenagers now that he had developed his own coping strategies and had his illness under control.

Coping with mental illness in some ways has more to do with addressing and enduring the stigma and discrimination that accompany it. That being said, how mental health consumers cope with stigma is a key factor in whether they recover. The coping strategies developed to deal with stigma and disempowerment are based in part on a desire not to be viewed simply as "taking" mental health services, but to be seen as giving something back as well (Wahl, 1999). The attitudes of the larger societal group participating in any reciprocal "giving" are critical to the ability of a person diagnosed with a mental illness to actively participate in the community and to achieve a sense of social reintegration. In addition, understanding the dynamic between those being stigmatized and those who are doing the stigmatizing may be important to our understanding of how to approach public education so as to help youth become more sympathetic and helpful toward their peers with mental illness.

It is crucial for each person to realize that mental illness is just a part of her experience—that it does not need to define her whole existence. It seems that the shift to self-acceptance frees youth to be accepted by others. Once their self-confidence returns, they are freer to explore the world again through "knowing" and "choosing" where they want to be. These, of course, are not easy tasks; rather, they are a lifelong pursuit—and with the appropriate interventions and social supports (especially peer), these young people have an opportunity to join and be a productive part of society.

Regarding the mental health needs of transitional youth, it is important to remember that adolescence and young adulthood are periods of transition and reorganization. As a result, it is critical to assess the mental health of adolescents and young adults in the context of the social determinants of health, which include the familial, social, and cultural expectations for age-appropriate thoughts, emotions, and behaviours (Health Canada, 1999a). Further, it is vital to understand the challenges faced by this age and stage if we are to fathom the enormous difficulties faced by young people with mental illnesses in their journeys of survival and achievement of identity, psychosocial development, and intimacy needs.

This is a critical time in transitional youths' psychosocial development as well as a critical time in the development of a mental illness. Adolescence is the peak age range for the onset of most major mental disorders (A. K. Malla, personal communication, December, 1999). Young people facing mental health problems could experience a permanent disruption in their ability to function (Kessler, Forster, Saunders, & Stang, 1995) because of the disruption of a serious illness with social and biological consequences. A major psychiatric disorder may disrupt adult identity formation so that the young person's efforts to achieve developmental milestones are permanently and negatively affected (McGorry et al., 1996).

Fear, lack of education, socio-cultural images (including advertising), and societal and economic competition all contribute to an untenable situation for a young person diagnosed with a mental illness. There is no more powerful barrier to success in society than the social stigma placed on individuals with a chronic illness that affects either social function or social identity (Goffman, 1963; Sontag, 1989). They alone must carry the burden of their loss, with no shield of protection. In their emotional and physiological states, they are truly vulnerable. Given the lived experience of youth with mental illness, controlling the effects of this reality and the resulting internal emotional state is often vital in their battle to regain a state of wellness. However, the resulting emotional effects of stigma may never be mediated or resolved, and this unfortunately can lead to a lifetime of constant struggle (Capponi, 1997).

These observations by researchers underscore the need for more quantitative and qualitative work in this area. It is particularly important to start with the lived experience of transitional youth. The findings presented in this book can be an important guide in understanding the internal and external worlds of individuals with mental health problems and how the mental health service system can support them in their growth and development.

To be effective, program development in the mental health system for youth must account for youth's experience and subjective interpretations of mental illness. As long as there are subjectively based meanings of mental illness for youth and subjective mechanisms for rationalizing and interpreting mental illness, programs based on health information data only and programs based on a rational, scientific medical model will not be adequate. When creating policy and programs, we must also consider the specific socio-cultural meanings of mental illness—for example, stigmatization and medicalization.

A gender-based analysis approach to policy, planning, and program development for mental health service delivery is significant in ensuring that we accurately tailor treatment to meet the needs of both male and female youth. As evidenced in the population studied, females tended to experience more internal, mood-related mental illnesses and were more concerned with their social standing than their male counterparts. Females were also typically more advanced developmentally. They were more concerned about employment, the future, and completing their education, and they were more likely in this study to be enrolled in a post-secondary program rather than a high school completion program. Males, on the other hand, were concerned about their family roles, had diagnoses that were more behavioural than those of females, and were more often in a high school completion program.

Though males and females experienced the illness itself and its social impacts differently, both reported benefiting from the youth-centred community psychosocial program from which they had been recruited. For example, the program focused on the social and vocational reintegration of youth and encouraged positive relationships between staff and clients that respected the client as full partner in goal setting. Participants stated that the opportunity to socialize and make friends was a key determinant in helping them adapt to mental illness and achieve and maintain a state of wellness or stabilization. Further, males and females stated that being treated as capable and having their choices respected was essential to boosting their self-confidence, reducing the effects of stigma, and achieving self-restoration and a positive self-image.

The mental health service system needs to continue to develop a mental health prevention and promotion approach. This public health approach, which involves community and media education, has the potential to influence people's attitudes toward mental illness by reducing their fear of the unknown and by helping them gain an understanding of treatment intervention and the needs of the population.

....

Limits and Benefits of This Research

■ THIS QUALITATIVE RESEARCH is limited in a number of ways. First, the results are not generalizable to all transition-aged youth with mental health problems, primarily due to the small sample size. Second, the three sites used were a convenience sample, since I knew of them through prior research and/or clinical work. The participants from the agencies dealing with youth and mental illness were specifically chosen because of their unique qualities and ability to identify experiences. Other limitations have to do with the researcher and participants. The quality of any research depends on the researcher's ability to build rapport, stay present, and remain faithful to the data being presented. As well, there may be limitations on my creative insight and ability to interpret and extract meaning from the data (Colaizzi, 1978).

Because this is a self-report study, the themes and analyses are limited by the participants' ability to retell their stories and by their capacity to describe their experiences with insight and accuracy. Further, while it is important to acknowledge that the corroborative experiences of the families and friends of transition-aged youth with mental health problems are important and often critical in understanding the "whole picture," this particular study is limited to the youth's experiences. This was a deliberate choice so that the voices of transition-aged youth could be heard and respected as valid.

The sample of interviewees is not intended to allow generalization about all youth with mental illness by class, occupation, education, race, age, or any other dimension. Instead, I have focused on the participants' subjective descriptions of their experiences of mental illness and on the developmental questions raised by these accounts. In this sense, the research does not lend itself to being generalizable to all youth with mental illness. Interpretations, then, are limited to this sample. In terms of generalizability, future studies will require the recruitment of a wider range of participants in greater numbers in order to compare results, analyze data, and determine the significance of emergence, loss, adaptation, and recovery to youth with mental health problems and their developmental and identity needs. Without further investigation, these results remain limited.

A benefit of qualitative research is that one can work with a small sample to extract the experience of individuals in specific populations and not only gain information (Colaizzi, 1978; Osborne, 1990; van Manen, 1990). Based on this assumption, this study has attempted to articulate the previously unknown experiences of a sample of transition-aged youth with mental health problems and compare the results with the available literature. Finally, a potential benefit of this study is that the information derived from exploring, describing, and explaining mental illness as experienced by transitional youth could contribute to a better understanding of the needs of youth and to youth-centred policy development; stimulate further research; and help with health planning for this population.

....

Suggestions for Future Research

■ FURTHER RESEARCH needs to be done to understand the reported 100% compliance rate for medication in this population to reveal the rationale. For example, is the importance of taking medication clinically significant or different in this age group for biological or social reasons in relation to the adult population? Could the compliance rate be because there are few alternative treatments available tailored to this specific population in relation to their adult counterparts? Could taking medication be a locus-of-control issue whereby this is the participants' only way to gain a sense of stability and therefore their only way to control her psychosocial needs?

Gender differences need further exploration to discover whether diagnostic criteria are applied differently to males versus females and whether systemic differences exist (Offord et al., 1987), and whether medications are prescribed differently, and if so, why (Leavey et al., 2008). Examples of differences in this research include the finding that after participants were formally assessed at a doctor's office or an emergency room, males were more likely to be admitted to a psychiatric ward in an acute care hospital and females were more likely to be sent home with or without (usually with) medication. This is an interesting finding that needs further investigation to determine whether the differences are warranted.

Given the average age of onset for participants, further investigation is needed to understand whether there is a relationship between biological hormonal changes and the age of onset of anxiety and/or depression in females. If a physiological relationship is found, could it account for some of the differences in the diagnostic labels between males and females? Following this line of investigation, further investigation is needed to see whether there are hormonal links between the onset of puberty in males and the types of diagnostic labels they receive, such as conduct disorder.

Conclusion

■ IN GENERAL, the existing literature regarding this population parallels what youth participants stated as their needs and experiences. Specifically, youth state they want appropriate and effective early intervention (in particular, medication) to help stabilize their illness so that they can concentrate on reclaiming their social and identity losses. When possible, staying with their families (as opposed to institutionalization) helped youth stabilize in their recovery and rehabilitation processes. Youth with mental illness face the same developmental challenges as their typical youth counterparts; however, they have much more difficulty in overcoming those challenges because of the biological and social impacts of the mental illness process (McGorry, 1992; McGorry et al., 1996). Stigma appears to be the greatest barrier facing youth with mental health problems.

Based on the findings of this study, it appears that health care providers, policy-makers, governments, and service systems need to begin addressing service delivery needs based in part on the psychosocial development of youth. That is, the provision of service needs to be developmentally focused so that youth can meet their life cycle needs by having the opportunity to rehabilitate, to get work-related training and education, and to have access to organized supports that include peer-related activities, groups, and programs. These peer groups need to provide advocacy, educate individuals and the community, and facilitate the recovery and reintegration processes of youth.

The identified gaps in service systems for youth with mental health problems need attention. The data clearly show that without formal peer support services for youth, the rest of the services seem less effective or important. It seems that when formal psychosocial supports and services with formalized peer components are available, more potential exists for youth to use these programs as an avenue of access to formal treatment interventions and as the basis for ongoing mental health and recovery. Further, there is inconsistent and insufficient information, data, research, and programming describing the needs of young people with mental illness. This research has begun to address the lack of data exploring and describing the lived experience of transition-aged youth with mental health problems.

Participants were able to tell their stories from their own perspectives. They shared developmental task and identity achievement challenges related to the disruption and interruption brought about by the onset of their mental illnesses. I developed the framework of emergence, loss, adaptation, and recovery based on the lived experiences of the participants, and this has provided a way to understand this group from a life cycle perspective. I sincerely hope that by interviewing these individuals, presenting their voices, and developing a theory for understanding the knowledge gained, this research will effect change for young people experiencing mental illness. By advancing the perception of mental illness from something to be feared or stigmatized to one of normalcy (in the sense of it [mental illness] being "just" another problem), I hope this research will help others understand that a diagnosis of mental illness can in fact be incorporated as part of daily living.

Finally, I hope these data will inspire future research and policy development, and improve service delivery in this very important area of helping young people achieve a healthy, productive, and balanced life.

Appendix

What was your experience of having been diagnosed with a mental health problem and/or illness and, living with that reality, how does it affect your life?

Questions

1. As a person diagnosed and living with a mental health problem/illness, can you tell me about your experience, as you would tell a story, a story that has a beginning, middle, and end?

2. Can you remember what it was like for you when you were first diagnosed with a mental health problem/illness?

3. What is it like for you now?

4. How did you (or someone else) first recognize that you had a problem?

5. What kind of issues did you have to face when first diagnosed?

6. What kind of issues do you face now?

7. What kind of personal changes (within you) have you experienced since being diagnosed?

8. What kinds of changes have happened (around you) in your life since becoming aware of your mental health problem/illness?

9. Can you describe how being diagnosed with a mental health problem has affected your:

   a) friendships/peer group

   b) family relationships

   c) independence from family of origin

   d) sexuality

   e) sense of self/identity

   f) academic pursuits

   g) career

10. Did you get the support you needed in getting help for your mental health problem/illness?

11. Did you experience anything helpful in your process?

12. Did you experience anything unhelpful in your process?

13. What parts of this story would you have liked to be different, if any?

14. If you were talking to another young person facing a diagnosis of a mental health problem/illness, what would you tell her/him?

References

Adaptation, *n*. (1999). *Merriam-Webster's collegiate dictionary* (10th ed.). Springfield, MA: Merriam-Webster.

American Foundation for Suicide Prevention. (2000). About suicide, facts. *American Foundation for Suicide Prevention Website*. Retrieved from http://www.afsp.org/index-1.htm

Aronson, E., Wilson, T. D., & Akert, R. M. (2005). *Social psychology* (5th ed.). Upper Saddle River, NJ: Prentice-Hall.

Becker, H. S. (1973). *Outsiders: Studies in the sociology of deviance.* New York, NY: Free Press.

Bettelheim, B. (1963). The problem of generations. In E. H. Erikson (Ed.), *Youth: Change and challenge.* New York, NY: Basic Books.

Biernat, M., & Dovidio, J. F. (2000). Stigma and stereotypes. In T. F. Heatherton, R. E. Kleck, M. R. Hebl, & J. G. Hull (Eds.), *The social psychology of stigma* (pp. 88–125). New York, NY: Guilford Press.

Booth, R. E., & Zhang, Y. (1997). Conduct disorder and HIV risk behaviors among runaway and homeless adolescents. *Drug and Alcohol Dependence, 48*(2), 69–76.

Brady, N. (1999). Mental illness hits one in five. *The Age,* 1.

Caine, V., & Boydell, K. M. (2010). Composing lives: Listening and responding to marginalized youth. *Education Canada, 50*(5), 42–45.

Cairney, J. (1998). Gender differences in the prevalence of depression among Canadian adolescents. *Canadian Journal of Public Health, 89*(3), 181–182.

Canadian Centre on Substance Abuse. (2013). *When mental health and substance abuse problems collide.* Retrieved from http://www.ccsa.ca/Resource%20Library/CCSA-Mental-Health -and-Substance-Abuse-2013-en.pdf

Canadian Institute for Health Information. (2007). *Improving the health of Canadians: Mental health and homelessness.* Ottawa: CIHI.

Canadian Mental Health Association, n.d. Fast facts about mental illness. Retrieved from http://www.cmha.ca/media/fast-facts-about-mental-illness/#.Us1uj7SmYk8

Canadian Mental Health Association, Ontario Division. (2000a). *Understanding stigma and mental health issues.* Retrieved from http://www.cmhawrb.on.ca/stigma.htm

Canadian Mental Health Association, Ontario Division. (2000b). *Understanding advocate: For child and youth mental health.* Retrieved from http://www.cmhawrb.on.ca/stigma.htm

Canadian Teachers' Federation. (2013). *Child and youth mental health.* Retrieved from www .ctf-fce.ca

Capponi, P. (1997). *Dispatches from the poverty line.* Toronto, ON: Penguin Books.

Cauce, A. M., Paradise, M., Embry, L., Morgan, C. J., Lohr, Y., Theofelis, J., Heger, J., & Wagner, V. (1998). Homeless youth in Seattle: Youth characteristics, mental health needs, and intensive case management. In M. H. Epstein, K. Kutash, and A. Duchnowski (Eds.), *Outcomes for children and youth with emotional and behavioral disorders and their families: Programs and evaluation best practices* (p. 738). Austin, TX: Pro-Ed.

Central Toronto Youth Services. (2002). *Community based youth mental health Program: A community-based psychosocial rehabilitation program for young adults with psychiatric disabilities, a program of Central Toronto Youth Services.* Toronto, ON: Central Toronto Youth Services.

Centre for Addiction and Mental Health. (1999). *Ontario Student Drug Study Use Survey.* Toronto, ON: Centre for Addiction and Mental Health.

Centres for Disease Control and Prevention. (2005). *Fact sheet: Suicide prevention-youth suicide.* Retrieved from http://www.cdc.gov/violenceprevention/pub/youth_suicide.html

Chen, L. P., Murad, M. H., Paras, M. L., Colbenson, K. M., Sattler, A. L., Goranson, E. N., Elamin, M. B., Seime, R. J., Shinozaki, G., Prokop, L. J., & Zirakzadeh, A. (2010). Sexual abuse and lifetime diagnosis of psychiatric disorders: Systematic review and meta-analysis. *Mayo Clinic Proceedings, 85*(7), 618–629.

Cheung, A. H., & Dewa, C. S. (2006). Canadian community health survey: Major depressive disorder and suicidality in adolescents. *Health Policy, 2*(2), 76–89.

Citizens for Public Justice. (2012). *Poverty trends scorecard.* Retrieved from http://www.cpj.ca/ files/docs/poverty-trends-scorecard.pdf

Clandinin, D. J., Steeves, P., Li, Y., Mickelson, J. R., Buck, G., Pearce, M., Caine, V., Lessard, S., Desrochers, C., Stewart, M., & Huber, M. (2010). Composing lives: A narrative account into the experiences of youth who left school early (Unpublished manuscript). Retrieved from http://www.elementaryed.ualberta.ca/~/media/elementaryed/Documents/Centres/CRTED/ComposingLives_FinalReport.pdf

Cohen, P., & Hesselbart, C. S. (1993). Demographic factors in the use of children's mental health services. *American Journal of Public Health, 83*, 49–52.

Colaizzi, P. F. (1978). Psychosocial research as the phenomenologist views it. In R. S. Valle & M. King (Eds.), *Existential-phenomenological alternatives for psychology* (pp. 48–71). New York, NY: Oxford University Press.

Craig, T. K., & Hodson, S. (1998). Homeless youth in London: Childhood antecedents and psychiatric disorder. *Psychological Medicine, 28*(6), 1379–1388.

Davidson, L. (2003). *Living outside mental illness: Qualitative studies of recovery in schizophrenia.* New York, NY: New York University Press.

Davidson, L., & Strauss, J. S. (1992). Sense of self in recovery from severe mental illness. *British Journal of Medical Psychology, 65*, 131–145.

Davis, M., & Vander-Stoep, A. (1996). *The transition to adulthood among adolescents who have serious emotional disturbance* (National Resource Center on Homelessness and Mental Illness). Delmar, NY: Policy Research Associates.

Dearing, E. (2008). Psychological costs of growing up poor. *Annals of the New York Academy of Sciences, 1136*, 324–332.

District Health Councils of Southwestern Ontario. (1996). *Southwest Region mental health – needs assessment (draft consultation document).* London, ON: Southwest Region, Mental Health Planners Working Group.

Early Psychosis Prevention and Intervention Centre. (2000). *Primary care project: EPPIC online.* Retrieved from http://avoca.vicnet.net.au/~eppic/primarycare.html

ECHRT (Egale Canada Human Rights Trust). (2013). *Report on outcomes and recommendations from the first national Lesbian, Gay, Bisexual, Trans, Two Spirit, Queer and Questioning (LGBTQ) Youth Suicide Prevention Summit 2012.* Egale Canada Human Rights Trust (ECHRT).

Egan, G. (1998). *The skilled helper* (6th ed.). Michigan: Brooks/Cole Publishing Company.

Emerson, R. M., Fretz, R. I., & Shaw, L. L. (1995). *Writing ethnographic field notes.* Chicago: University of Chicago Press.

Erikson, E. H. (Ed.). (1963). *Youth: Change and challenge.* New York, NY: Basic Books.

Erikson, E. H. (1968). *Identity: Youth and crisis.* New York, NY: W.W. Norton & Co.

Erikson, E. H. (1980). *Identity and the life cycle.* Toronto, ON: W.W. Norton & Co.

Erikson, E. H. (1999). Identity: Youth and crisis. In J. Kaplan (Ed.), *Using literature to help troubled teenagers cope with identity issues* (pp. 1–22). Westport, CT: Greenwood Press.

Eskin, M. (1995). Suicidal behavior as related to social support and assertiveness among Swedish and Turkish high school students: A cross-cultural investigation. *Journal of Clinical Psychology, 51*(2), 158–172.

Family Service Toronto. (2011) *Revisiting family security in insecure times: 2011 report card on child and family poverty in Canada.* Toronto, ON: Family Service Toronto.

Fassler, D. (2000). A common sense 10-point plan to address the problem of school violence. *American Academy of Child and Adolescent Psychiatry.* Retrieved from http://www.aacap .org/whatsnew/10point.htm

Firsten, T. (1991). Violence in the lives of women of psychiatric wards. *Canadian Women Studies / Les Cahiers de la Femme, 11*(4), 45–48.

Frankish, C. J., Hwang, S. W., & Quantz, D. (2005). Homelessness and health in Canada. *Canadian Journal of Public Health, 96,* S23–S29.

Freyers, T., Melzer, D., & Jenkins, R. (2003). Social inequalities and the common mental disorders. *Social Psychiatry and Psychiatric Epidemiology, 38*(5), 229–237.

Glaser, B. G., & Strauss, A. L. (1967). *The discovery of grounded theory: Strategies for qualitative research.* New York, NY: Aldine De Gruyter.

Goffman, E. (1963). *Stigma: Notes on the management of spoiled identity.* Englewood Cliffs, NJ: Prentice-Hall.

Goffman, E. (1967). *Interaction ritual: Essays on face-to-face behaviour.* New York, NY: Pantheon Books.

Goffman, E. (1974). *Frame analysis: An essay on the organization of experience.* Cambridge, MA: Harvard University Press.

Gove, W. R., & Herb, T. R. (1974). Stress and mental illness among the young: A comparison of the sexes. *Social Forces, 53*(2), 256–265.

Government of Canada. (2006). *The human face of mental health and mental illness in Canada.* Ottawa, ON: Government of Canada.

Gulliver, A., Griffiths, K. M., & Christensen, H. (2010). Perceived barriers and facilitators to mental health help-seeking in young people: A systematic review. *BMC Psychiatry, 10*(113). Retrieved from http://www.biomedcentral.com/1471-244X/10/113

Hale, N. (1980). Freud's reflections on work and love. In N. J. Smelser & E. H. Erikson (Eds.), *Themes of love and work in adulthood* (pp. 29–41). Cambridge, MA: Harvard University Press.

Hamid-Balma, S. (2005). Suicide 101: The statistics of risk. *Visions, 2*(7), 6–7.

Health Canada. (1997a). Meeting the needs of youth-at-risk in Canada: Learnings from a national community development project. Minister of Public Works and Government Services Canada. (Cat. #H39-411/1997E). Ottawa, ON: Health Canada.

Health Canada. (1997b). *Meeting the needs of youth-at-risk in Canada: Learnings from a national community development project.* Ottawa, ON: Ministry of Public Works and Government Services Canada.

Health Canada. (1999a). *Toward a healthy future: Second report on the health of Canadians.* Ottawa, ON: Federal, Provincial, and Territorial Advisory Committee on Population Health.

Health Canada. (1999b). *Statistical report on the health of Canadians.* Ottawa, ON: Federal, Provincial, and Territorial Advisory Committee on Population Health.

Health Canada. (2011). *Canadian alcohol and drug use monitoring survey.* Retrieved from http://www.hc-sc.gc.ca/hc-ps/drugs-drogues/stat/_2011/summary-sommaire-eng.php

Health Canada (2012). *Canadian tobacco use monitoring survey 2012.* Retrieved from http://www.hc-sc.gc.ca/hc-ps/tobac-tabac/research-recherche/stat/ctums-esutc_2012-eng.php

Heatherton, T. F., Kleck, R. E., Hebl, M. R., & Hull, J. G. (Eds.). (2000). *The social psychology of stigma.* New York, NY: Guilford Press.

Hilton, C., Osborn, M., & Serjent, G. (1997). Psychiatric disorder in young adults in Jamaica. *International Journal of Social Psychiatry, 43*(4), 257–268.

Holmes, G. (1995). *Helping teenagers into adulthood: A guide for the next generation.* Westport, CT: Greenwood Publishing Group.

hooks, b. (2000a). *Feminist theory: From margin to center* (2nd ed.). Cambridge, MA: South End Press.

hooks, b. (2000b). *Where we stand: Class matters.* New York, NY: Routledge.

Illich, I. (1976). *Limits to medicine: Medical nemesis: The expropriation of health.* New York, NY: Penguin Books.

Jane-Llopis, E., & Matytsina, I. (2006). Mental health and alcohol, drugs and tobacco: A review of the comorbidity between mental disorders and the use of alcohol, tobacco and illicit drugs. *Drug and Alcohol Review, 25*(6), 515–536.

Kessler, R. C., Chiu, W. T., Demler, O., & Walters, E. E. (2006). Prevalence, severity, and comorbidity of twelve-month DSM-IV disorders in the National Comorbidity Survey Replication (NCS-R). *Archives of General Psychiatry, 62*(6), 617–627.

Kessler, R. C., Forster, C. L., Saunders, W. B., & Stang, P. E. (1995). Consequences of psychiatric disorders: Educational attainment. *American Journal of Psychiatry, 152*, 1026–1032.

Kilpatrick, D. G., Acierno, R., Saunders, B. E., Resnick, H. S., Best, C. L., & Schnurr, P. P. (2000). Risk factors for adolescent substance abuse and dependence: Data from a national sample. *Journal of Consulting and Clinical Psychology, 68*, 19–30.

Kirby, M. J. L., & Keon, W. J. (2006). *Out of the shadows at last: Transforming mental health, mental illness and addiction services in Canada: Final report of The Standing Senate Committee on Social Affairs, Science and Technology.* Ottawa, ON: Standing Senate Committee on Social Affairs, Science and Technology.

Klee, H., & Reid, P. (1998). Drug use among the young homeless: Coping through self-medication. *Health, 2*(2), 115–134.

Kutcher, S., & McLuckie, A. (2011). Evergreen: A child and youth mental health framework for Canada. *Paediatrics & Child Health, 16*(7), 388.

Kutcher, S. P., & Szumilas, M. (2008). Youth suicide prevention. *Canadian Medical Association Journal, 178*(3), 282–285.

Lasch, C. (1979). *The culture of narcissism.* Toronto, ON: George J. McLeod.

Lasch, C. (1984). *The minimal self: Psychic survival in troubled times.* New York, NY: W.W. Norton & Company.

Lau, R. W. (1994). Fatal suicides among children and adolescents 1992–1994. *Bulletin of the Hong Kong Psychological Society, 32–33*, 105–112.

Leavey, J. E. (2003). *The meaning of mental illness to youth.* (doctoral dissertation). Toronto, ON: University of Toronto.

Leavey, J. E. (2005). Youth experiences of living with mental health problems: Emergence, loss, adaptation and recovery (ELAR). *Canadian Journal of Community Mental Health, 24*(2), 109–126.

Leavey, J. E. (2011). When youth know about their mental disorder before caregivers do: Youth-identified duration of untreated mental disorder (YIDUMD). *Psychosis, 3*, 86–89.

Leavey, J. E, Flexhaug, M., & Ehmann, T. (2008). Review of the literature regarding early intervention for children and adolescents aged 0–15 experiencing a first-episode psychiatric disturbance. *Early Intervention Psychiatry, 2*(4), 212–224.

Leavey, J. E., Goering, P., Macfarlane, D., Bradley, S., & Cochrane, J. (2000). *The gap: Moving toward youth-centred mental health care for transitional aged youth (16–24).* Toronto, ON: Health Systems Research and Consulting Unit, Centre for Addiction and Mental Health.

Levinson, D. J. (1980). Toward a conception of the adult life course. In N. J. Smelser & E. H. Erikson (Eds.), *Themes of work and love in adulthood* (pp. 265–290). Cambridge, MA: Harvard University Press.

Lincoln, C. V., & McGorry, P. (1995). Who cares? Pathways to psychiatric care for young people experiencing a first episode of psychosis. *Psychiatric Services, 46*(11), 1166–1171.

Lorber, J. (1997). *Gender and the social construction of illness.* Thousand Oaks, CA: Sage Publications.

Lynskey, M. T., & Fergusson, D. M. (1997). Factors protecting against the development of adjustment difficulties in youth adults exposed to childhood sexual abuse. *Child Abuse and Neglect, 21*(12), 1177–1190.

Macnaughton, E. (1997). Early psychosis intervention in Canada. *Visions: BC Mental Health Journal.* Retrieved from http://www.cmha-bc.org/visions/vsum 97c.html

Macnaughton, E. (1999). *The BC early intervention study: Report of findings.* Vancouver, BC: Canadian Mental Health Association (British Columbia Division).

Mahoney, M. J. (1991). *Human change processes: The scientific foundations of psychotherapy.* New York, NY: Basic Books.

Malla, A. K. (1999). When should drug treatment be initiated in schizophrenia? *Journal of Psychiatry & Neuroscience, 24*(4), 363.

Malla, A.K., & Norman, R. M. G. (1999). Facing the challenges of intervening early in psychosis. *Annals RCPSC, 32*(7), 394–397.

Malla, A. K., Norman, R. M. G., & Voruganti, L. P. (1999). Improving outcome in schizophrenia: The case for early intervention. *Canadian Medical Association Journal, 160*(6), 843–846. Retrieved from http://www.cma.ca/cmaj/vol-160/issue-6/0843.htm

Marcia, J. (1966). Development and validation of ego identity status. *Journal of Personality and Social Psychology, 3*, 551–558.

Masten, A. S. (2004). Regulatory processes, risk, and resilience in adolescent development. *Annals of the New York Academy of Sciences, 1021*, 310–310.

McCreary Centre Society. (1999). *Healthy connections: Listening to BC youth.* Burnaby, BC: McCreary Centre Society.

McGorry, P. D. (1992). The concept of recovery and secondary prevention in psychotic disorders. *Australian and New Zealand Journal of Psychiatry, 26*, 3–17.

McGorry, P. D. (1995). Psychoeducation in first-episode psychosis: A therapeutic process. *Psychiatry, 58*, 313–328.

McGorry, P. D., Edwards, J., Mihalopoulos, C., Harrigan, S. M., & Jackson, H. J. (1996). EPPIC: An evolving system of early detection and optimal management. *Schizophrenia Bulletin, 22*(2), 305–326.

McGorry, P. D., Killackey, E., & Yung, A. (2008). Early intervention in psychosis: Concepts, evidence and future directions. *World Psychiatry, 7*(3), 148–156.

McLean, C. P., Asnaani, A., Litz, B. T., & Hofmann, S. G. (2011). Gender differences in anxiety disorders: Prevalence, course of illness, comorbidity and burden of illness. *Journal of Psychiatric Research, 45*(8), 1027–35.

McLeod, J., & Shanahan, M. J. (1993). Poverty, parenting, and children's mental health. *American Sociological Review, 58*(3), 351–366.

Merikangas, K., R., He, J., Burstein, M., Swanson, S., A., Avenevoli, S., Cui, L., Benjet, C., Georgiades, K., & Swendsen, J. (2010). Lifetime prevalence of mental disorders in U.S. adolescents: Results from the National Comorbidity Study-Adolescent Supplement (NCS-A). *Journal of the American Academy of Child and Adolescent Psychiatry, 49*(10), 980–989.

Miller, C. T., & Major, B. (2000). Coping with stigma and prejudice. In T. F. Heatherton, R. E. Kleck, M. R. Hebl, & J. G. Hull (Eds.), *The social psychology of stigma* (pp. 243–272). New York, NY: Guilford Press.

Ministry of Health, Ontario. (1993). *Putting people first.* Toronto, ON: Queen's Printer for Ontario.

Ministry of Health, Ontario. (2000). *2000 and beyond: Strengthening Ontario's mental health system: A report on the consultative review of mental health reform in the province of Ontario.* Retrieved from http://www.gov.on.ca/MOH/english/pub/mental/mentalreform.html

Moller, M. D., & Murphy, M. F. (1997). The three R's rehabilitation program: A prevention approach for the management of relapse symptoms associated with psychiatric diagnoses. *Journal of Psychiatric Rehabilitation, 20*(3), 42–48.

Moller, M. D., & Murphy, M. F. (1998). *Recovering from psychosis: A wellness approach.* USA: Psychiatric Rehabilitation Nurses.

Morrow, M., & Chappell, M. (1999). *Hearing voices: Mental health care for women.* Vancouver, BC: BC Centre of Excellence for Women's Health.

Murphy, M. F., & Moller, M. D. (1996). The three R's program: A wellness approach to rehabilitation of neurobiological disorders. *International Journal of Psychiatric Nursing Research, 3*(1), 308–317.

National Early Psychosis Program. (1997). Early psychosis activities Australia-wide. Retrieved from http://ariel.ucs.unimelb.edu.au/~nepp

National Institute of Mental Health. (1990). *The stigma of mental illness* (Publication no. [ADM] 90-1470). Washington, DC: U.S. Department of Health and Human Services.

National Learning Community on Youth Homelessness. (2013). Mental health of homeless youth. *2013 Mental Health eBulletin.* Retrieved from http://learningcommunity.ca/lcwp/tags/mental-health-of-homeless-youth

Navaneelan, T. (2012). *Suicide rates: An overview.* (Statistics Canada Catalogue no. 82-624-x). Retrieved from http://www.statcan.gc.ca/pub/82-624-x/2012001/article/11696-eng.htm

Neuberg, S. L., Smith, D. M., & Asher, T. (2000). Why people stigmatize: Toward a biocultural framework. In T. F. Heatherton, R. E. Kleck, M. R. Hebl, & J. G. Hull (Eds.), *The social psychology of stigma* (pp. 31–61). New York, NY: Guilford Press.

Neuman, B. (1982). *The Neuman Systems Model: Application to nursing education and practice.* Norwalk, CT: Appleton-Century-Crofts.

Neuman, B. (1996). The Neuman Systems Model in research and practice. *Nursing Science Quarterly, 9*(2), 67–70.

Offord, D. R., Boyle, M. H., Szatmari, P., Rae-Grant, N. I., Links, P. S., Cadman, D. T., Byles, J. A., Crawford, J. W., Blum, H. M., Byrne, C., Thomas, H., & Woodward, C. A. (1987). Ontario child health study II: Six-month prevalence of disorder and rates of service utilization. *Archives of General Psychiatry, 44*, 832–836.

Ogrodnik, L. (2008). *Child and youth victims of police-reported Crime, 2008.* Retrieved from http://www.statcan.gc.ca/pub/85f0033m/85f0033m2010023-eng.pdf

Osborne, J. W. (1990). Some basic existential-phenomenological research methodology for counsellors. *Canadian Journal of Counselling, 24*, 79–91.

Paglia-Boak, A., Adlaf, E. M., Hamilton, H. A., Beitchman, J. H., Wolfe, F., & Mann, R. E. (2012). *The mental health and well-being of Ontario students, 1991–2011.* Detailed OSDUHS findings (CAMH Research Document Series, No. 34). Toronto, ON: Centre for Addiction and Mental Health.

Papalia, D. E., & Olds, S. W. (1981). *Human development* (2nd ed.). New York, NY: McGraw-Hill.

Patel, V., Flisher, A. J., Hetrick, S. E., & McGorry, P. D. (2007). Mental health of young people: A global public-health challenge. *Lancet, 369*, 1302–1313.

Public Health Agency of Canada. (2006). *The human face of mental health and mental illness in Canada.* Ottawa: Minister of Public Works and Government Services Canada.

Rice, M. J., & Moller, M. D. (2006). Wellness outcomes of group psychoeducation on trauma and abuse. *Archives of Psychiatric Nursing, 20*, 94–102.

Rich, C. L., & Runeson, B. S. (1995). Mental illness and youth suicide. *American Journal of Psychiatry, 152*(8), 1239–1240.

Rudolph, K. D., Lambert, S. F., Clark, A. G., & Kurlakowsky, K. D. (2001). Negotiating the transition to middle school: The role of self-regulatory processes. *Child Development, 72*(3), 929–960.

Santor, D. A., Kusumakar, V., Poulin, C., and LeBlanc, J. C. (2007). Online health promotion, early identification of difficulties, and help seeking in young people. *Journal of the American Academy of Child and Adolescent Psychiatry, 46*(1), 50–59.

Santor, D., Short, K., & Ferguson, B. (2009). *Taking mental health to school: A policy-oriented paper on school-based mental health for Ontario.* The provincial Centre of Excellence for Child and Youth Mental Health at CHEO. Retrieved from http://www.excellenceforchild-andyouth.ca/sites/default/files/position_sbmh.pdf

Schwab-Stone, M. E., & Briggs-Gowan, M. J. (1998). The scope and prevalence of psychiatric disorders in childhood and adolescence. In International Association for Child and Adolescent Psychiatry and Allied Professions (Ed.), *Designing mental health services and systems for children and adolescents: A shrewd investment.* Philadelphia, PA: Brunner/Mazel.

Silverman, A. B., Reinherz, H. Z., & Giaconia, R. M. (1996). The long-term sequelae of child and adolescent abuse: A longitudinal community study. *Child Abuse and Neglect, 20*(8), 709–723.

Smelser, N. J., & Erikson, E. H. (Eds.). (1980). *Themes of work and love in adulthood.* Cambridge, MA: Harvard University Press.

Smyth, J. (2013). Young people speaking back from the margins, in youth, education, and marginality. In K. Tilleczek and H. B. Ferguson (Eds.), *Local and Global Expressions.* Toronto: Sick Kids Community and Mental Health.

Sontag, S. (1977). Photography unlimited. *New York Review, 23*, 26–31.

Sontag, S. (1978). *Illness as metaphor.* New York, NY: Farrar, Straus and Giroux.

Sontag, S. (1989). *AIDS and its metaphors.* New York, NY: Anchor Books, Doubleday.

Standing Senate Committee on Social Affairs, Science and Technology. (2006). *Out of the shadows at last: Transforming mental health, mental illness and addiction services in Canada.* Ottawa, ON: Standing Senate Committee on Social Affairs, Science and Technology.

Statistics Canada and Health Canada. (2000). *Canadian tobacco use monitoring survey (CTUM).* Ottawa, ON: Statistics Canada and Health Canada.

Statistics Canada. (2003). Canadian Community Health Survey—Mental health and well-being. *The Daily*, Statistics Canada.

Statistics Canada. (2012). *Suicide and suicide rate, by sex and by age group.* Retrieved from http://www.statcan.gc.ca/tables-tableaux/sum-som/l01/cst01/hlth66a-eng.htm

Stover, L. T., & Hopkins, J. R. (1999). Identity within the family. In J. Kaplan (Ed.), *Using literature to help troubled teenagers cope with identity issues* (pp. 1–22). Westport, CT: Greenwood Press.

Strauss, A. L., & Corbin, J. (1990). *Qualitative analysis for social scientists.* New York: Cambridge University Press.

Strauss, A. L., & Corbin, J. (1994). Grounded Theory methodology: An overview. In N. K. Denzin & Y. S. Lincoln (Eds.), *Handbook of qualitative research.* Thousand Oaks, CA: Sage Publications.

Strauss, A. L., & Corbin, J. (1998). *Basics of qualitative research: Techniques and procedures for developing grounded theory* (2nd ed.). Thousand Oaks, CA: Sage Publications.

Thames Valley District Health Council. (1997). *System design for mental health reform in the Thames Valley district*. London, ON: Thames Valley District Health Council.

Tilleczek, K., & Ferguson, B. (2007). *Elementary to secondary school: A review of selected literature*. Community Health Systems Resource Group, The Hospital for Sick Children for the Ontario Ministry of Education.

Tipper, J. (1997). *The Canadian girl-child: Determinants of the health and well-being of girls and young women*. Ottawa, ON: Canadian Institute of Child Health.

Ungar, M., & Teram, E. (2000). Drifting toward mental health: High-risk adolescents and the process of empowerment. *Youth Society, 32*(2), 228–252.

Unger, K. V., Anthony, W. A., Sciarappa, K., & Rogers, E. S. (1991). A supported education program for young adults with long-term mental illness. *Hospital and Community Psychiatry, 42*(8), 838–842.

Unger, J. B., Kipke, M. D., Simon, T. R., Montgomery, S. B., & Johnson, C. J. (1997). Homeless youths and young adults in Los Angeles: Prevalence of mental health problems and the relationship between mental health and substance abuse disorders. *American Journal of Community Psychology, 25*(3), 371–394.

U.S. Department of Health and Human Services. (1999). *Mental health: A report of the surgeon general*. Rockville, MD: U.S. Department of Health and Human Services, Substance use and Mental Health Services Administration, Center for Mental Health Services, National Institutes of Health, National Institute of Mental Health.

van Manen, M. (1990). *Researching lived experience*. Ann Arbor, MI: Althouse Press.

Vancouver/Richmond Health Board. (1998). *Mental health services for youth: Where are they? A report of the findings and recommendations of the Children and Youth Population Health Advisory Committee*. Vancouver, BC: Vancouver/Richmond Health Board.

Vega, W. A., Aguilar-Gaxiola, A. S. L., Bijl, R., Borges, G., Caraveo-Anduaga, J. J., DeWit, D. J., Heeringa, S. G., Kessler, R. C., Kolody, B., Merikangas, K. R., Molnar, B. E., Walters, E. E., Warner, L. A., & Wittchen, H. U. (2002). Prevalence and age of onset for drug use in seven international sites: Results from the international consortium of psychiatric epidemiology. *Drug and Alcohol Dependence, 68*(3), 285–297.

Waddell, C., & Shepherd, C. (2002). Prevalence of Mental Disorders in Children and Youth. Mental Health Evaluation and Community Consultation Unit: University of British Columbia. Retrieved from http://www.mcf.gov.bc.ca/mental_health/pdf/02a_cymh.pdf

Wade, T. J., Cairney, J., & Pevalin, D. J. (2002). Emergence of gender differences in depression during adolescence: National panel results from three countries. *Journal of the American Academy of Child & Adolescent Psychiatry, 41*(2), 190–198.

Wahl, O. F. (1999). *Telling is risky business: Mental health consumers confront stigma.* New Brunswick, NJ: Rutgers University Press.

Ward, A. J. (1992). Adolescent suicide and other self-destructive behaviours: Adolescent attitude survey data and interpretation. *Residential Treatment for Children and Youth, 9*(3), 49–64.

World Health Organization. (2001). *Mental health: Strengthening mental health promotion.* Geneva, Switzerland: WHO.

Wilson, P. (1995). Working space: A mentally healthy youth nation. *Youth and Policy, 51* (Winter), 60–63.

Index

of social identity, 2, 56; sociological/
psychosocial perspectives on identity,
32–33
self-acceptance, 155
self-confidence: and bullying, 39
self-esteem: effect of media images on,
71–73; restoration of, 32, 100, 111
self-evaluation, 32
self-harming behaviours, 28, 61–62, 114–15
self-marginalization, 2, 17–18, 76–77
self-surveillance, 21
service delivery needs: considerations for
practice, 130; developmental focus on,
4–5, 31; gap in service to youth, 26,
57, 65–67, 145–46, 160; for recovery,
136; youth-focused mental health
initiatives, 146–48
severe emotional disturbance (SED):
definition, 26; prevalence of, 26–27
sexual abuse: association with mental
illness, 35; in history of research
participants, 47, 48
sexuality: and adult identity development,
29, 34, 58, 78; ambivalence toward
intimate relationships, 86–87; dating,
and interrupted sexual development,
89–92; expression of, 22. See also
LGBTQ youth
social acceptance, 76–77
social barriers: and chronic illness, 149
social class: effect on treatment options,
20–21; and transition to adulthood, 28
social determinants of health:
consideration of in assessment

process, 153–54; work, and economic
stability, 33, 139–41
social dysfunction, 37
social frameworks: as guided doings, 10–12
social identity, 31–33, 149
social integration: and role of group
behaviour, 9
social standing: and interrupted social
development, 86–88; loss of, 2, 78,
83–84
social stigma. See stigma
social supports: withdrawal of, 86
social withdrawal: behavioural expression
of, 16
Sontag, Susan, 9, 149, 156; "citizens of
illness" and, 132; demonization of the
ill, 19; on metaphors, 18–19; stigma of
the ill, 14–15; process of illness, 131;
and "self-surveillance," 21
speed, 37
spoiled identity, 21; avoidance of, 9;
internalized stigma of, 75; as label, 14;
pre-illness sense of self, 135
stabilization, 4; and adaptation, 56–57, 58;
adjustment, 106; correct medication,
101–2; improvement in daily living
activities, 103–4; through medication,
80–81, 97–99
statistical reporting: inconsistencies in, 27
Standing Senate Committee on Social
Affairs, Science and Technology, 26,
27, 174
Statistics Canada: Canadian Community
Health Survey, 37–38; depression